EMDR and the

Art of Psychotherapy

With Children

Treatment Manual

D1605113

About the Authors

Robbie Adler-Tapia, PhD, is a licensed psychologist who has worked with traumatized children and their families for more than 25 years. Dr. Adler-Tapia is EMDRIA certified in EMDR, an EMDRIA approved consultant, an EMDR Institute Facilitator, and an EMDR HAP trainer-in-training and has volunteered for EMDR HAP in New Orleans. Dr. Adler-Tapia has extensive training in developmental psychology and working with children 0–3 years of age. Dr. Adler-Tapia has served as clinical director for several nonprofit agencies and is currently in private practice in Tempe, Arizona, and has taught graduate-level classes on counseling and consultation. Dr. Adler-Tapia provides counseling, consultation, and psychological services for children and families referred by Arizona Child Protective Services and works with local police departments providing counseling and CISD services at her private office in Tempe. Dr. Adler-Tapia has provided training internationally on psychotherapy with traumatized children, including specialized trauma treatment with EMDR at several EMDRIA conferences, and she is conducting research on EMDR with young children. With her colleague Carolyn Settle, MSW, LCSW, Dr. Adler-Tapia is coauthor of *EMDR Treatment Manual: Children's Protocol* and has coauthored several studies on EMDR with children.

Carolyn Settle, MSW, LCSW, is EMDRIA certified in EMDR, is an EMDRIA approved consultant, an EMDR Institute Facilitator, and an EMDR HAP trainer-in-training. Carolyn has been an EMDR facilitator for 11 years and has facilitated in Japan, as part of the HAP team in New Orleans, and for the psychiatric residents at the University of Pittsburgh. Carolyn also provides specialty training on EMDR for children and has presented at several EMDRIA conferences and on using EMDR with children at EMDR Europe. Carolyn is a clinical social worker with 30 years of experience working with children. Carolyn specializes in posttraumatic stress disorder, depression, anxiety, phobias, attention-deficit/hyperactivity disorder, and gifted counseling for children, adolescents, and adults in her private practice in Scottsdale, Arizona. Along with her colleague Dr. Adler-Tapia, Ms. Settle has conducted a fidelity study on using EMDR with children under 10 years of age.

EMDR and the Art of Psychotherapy With Children Treatment Manual

Robbie Adler-Tapia, PhD   Carolyn Settle, MSW, LCSW

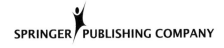

SPRINGER PUBLISHING COMPANY

New York

Springer Publishing Company, LLC
11 West 42nd Street
New York, NY 10036
www.springerpub.com

Acquisitions Editor: Sheri W. Sussman
Production Editor: Julia Rosen
Cover design: Joanne E. Honigman
Composition: Apex CoVantage

08 09 10 11 12/ 5 4 3 2 1

ISBN: 978-0-8261-1119-7

Printed in the United States of America by Book-Mart Press.

Contents

Introduction to the Manual

This manual is based on EMDR theory created by Dr. Francine Shapiro and documented in Dr. Shapiro's books (1995, 2001). We have written this treatment manual to provide a simple and practical way to use EMDR in psychotherapy with children and adolescents. The EMDR scripts, protocols, and forms that were detailed in the book *EMDR and the Art of Psychotherapy With Children,* also written by the authors of this manual. The manual was derived from the *EMDR Fidelity Research Manual* for children, also created by these authors. By using a standard treatment protocol for providing EMDR psychotherapy for children and by conducting pre- and post-treatment assessments, therapists can also conduct their own study of treatment outcomes. In addition to contributing to research, this manual is beneficial to the therapist and the client in order to monitor treatment progress and outcomes.

The manual is organized consistent with the chapters in the book and begins with the directions to the therapist, session protocols, therapist's scripts, and forms for each phase of the protocol. Instructions to the therapist provide an overview of the goals for the specific phase of EMDR with suggestions for case conceptualization. Session protocols include the steps for the specific phase of treatment. Next we have provided therapist's scripts that include possible wording for the therapist to use with the child, set in italics. The final section of each phase includes forms as templates for the therapist to use for documentation and case planning.

For the purposes of this treatment manual, the reader will note that the terms *child* and *parent* are used to refer to the client and the client's parent or caretaker. The session protocols are suggested guidelines; however, the timing of the individual sessions is tailored to the individual child and parent needs.

When using the EMDR protocol with clients of any age, but especially with children, the therapist can integrate techniques and tools from play therapy, art therapy, sand tray therapy, and any other techniques the therapist determines helpful for clients to express themselves.

The forms in this *Manual* are available to all purchasers. Please go to www. springerpub.com/adlerforms. After you download the file, you can access the forms by entering the password ADLER1.

Section 1

Client History and Treatment Planning Phase

This section relates to chapter 3 of the book, *EMDR and the Art of Psychotherapy With Children.*

Instructions to the Therapist for Client History and Treatment Planning

With Phase 1 of EMDR, Client History and Treatment Planning, begins the process of becoming attuned with the client's unique concerns and issues and physical and emotional capacities and creating the safety necessary for clients to process trauma. Pacing the use of EMDR is an important part of the therapist's role of attuning himself or herself to client physical and emotional presentation and needs, and preparing the client for EMDR. Special emphasis should be placed on assessing the child's age, developmental level, and understanding of the context of the child's life experiences in order to guide the treatment process. The therapist should *also* attend to the child's nonverbal communication, including changes in breathing, mannerisms, skin tone, and so on during treatment. The child's ability to tolerate affect also needs to be assessed. In addition, the therapist should assess the child's current stability. Assessment of the child's current stability should include evaluation of any risk of suicidal behaviors and/or whether a child is medically fragile. Children who are currently not stable may require more time spent in the Preparation Phase as is discussed in chapter 4 of *EMDR and the Art of Psychotherapy With Children.*

Evaluating targets also begins as you take the child's history. It does not mean that you have identified the specific targets for processing at this point, but that you make notes, mental or written, to explore the possible target issues and negative beliefs as you proceed.

The therapist begins the Client History and Treatment Planning process by completing the Client History and Treatment Planning Forms. When it is time for the Target Identification Process, the child is asked to wait in the playroom while the parent is interviewed. Deciding not to have the child in the office while interviewing the parent is for several reasons: First, the parent may have his or her own issues and unresolved affect related to the incidents, which will be identified for the child. Second, the parent's targets may be different from the child's, and we do not want the parent's statements to contaminate what the child may report. If the child listens to the parent's statements, the child may echo the parent's statements rather than reporting the child's own issues/targets. The parent's idea or beliefs about targets for the child may be different from those of the child. However, the child might not volunteer targets that are embarrassing, or the child may have forgotten a target that needs to be addressed in treatment. All of these issues need to be considered by the therapist; yet ultimately, the target selected must resonate for the child. We suggest that the therapist interview the parent for possible targets while the child waits in an adjacent room or consider having the child not attend this session.

This protocol describes session guidelines; however, the amount of information to be included in each session depends on the unique needs of the child and family. This process is explained in great deal in chapter 3 of the book, *EMDR and the Art of Psychotherapy With Children*. It is possible to integrate the Mapping and Graphing techniques to identify targets starting from the Client History and Treatment Planning Phase of EMDR.

Session Protocol for Client History and Treatment Planning

1. Prior to or at the first session of EMDR the parent receives and completes:

   • Informed Consent for Treatment

   • Informed Assent for Treatment (to be signed by child)

   • Health Insurance Portability and Accountability Act (HIPAA) (For therapists practicing in the United States)

   • Additional paperwork as indicated by the therapist's professional, agency, and/or governmental guidelines

2. The therapist greets and introduces himself or herself to the child and parent.

3. The therapist reviews the Initial Patient Information Packet and all Informed Consent forms. The therapist explains psychotherapy and reviews the forms with parents and children. The therapist then answers child and parent questions.

4. The parent participates in the intake process per the professional and/or agency's intake procedures.

5. The parent completes the Intake Form for Child/Adolescent Psychotherapy.

6. The parent participates in the Child/Adolescent Intake Interview with the therapist.

7. The child participates in the Child/Adolescent Intake Interview.

8. The therapist contacts other providers, including pediatrician or primary care physician, psychiatrist, therapists, or other medical/mental health providers.

9. The therapist has parent(s) sign appropriate release of information forms.

10. The therapist contacts other professionals including school and day care.

11. The therapist requests other assessment, testing, or additional records that would assist in treatment planning.

12. The therapist provides the parent with self-report instruments and explains the purpose of the instruments. The parent is instructed to complete the Behavioral Assessment System for Children (2nd ed., Reynolds & Kamphaus, 2004; BASC-2), Children's Dissociative Checklist, Version 3 (CDC3; Putnam, 1997), or the Adolescent Dissociative Experiences Scale (A-DES; Armstrong et al., 1997) Sensory Integration Checklist, and Traumatic Stress Checklist for Infants and Toddlers, Preschoolers (if child is less than 8 years; Adler-Tapia, 2000) and return forms to the therapist. (See chapter 3 in *EMDR and the Art of Psychotherapy With Children* for detailed information and references for assessment tools.)

13. The therapist reviews assessment forms with the parent as appropriate. If the child is over 8, the therapist will complete Trauma Symptom Checklist for Children (TSCC; Briere, 1996) with the client in the first session. The parent is also asked to have the teacher/caregiver complete BASC-2 Teacher Format and return the forms at the next session.

14. The therapist completes the Children's Impact of Traumatic Events Scale-Revised (CITES-R; Wolfe et al., 1991) or *The Child's Reaction to Traumatic Events Scale-Revised* (CRTES-Revised; Jones, Fletcher, & Ribbe, 2002) and TSCC with the child in the therapy session.

15. The therapist completes the Client History and Treatment Planning using forms provided. (Client History and Treatment Planning process is completed with the child and parent in session except where indicated on the form.)

16. The therapist begins to note possible targets for EMDR based on presenting problems suggested by the child and parent to assist in case conceptualization.

17. The therapist uses targets identified to create a targeting sequence for use in the Assessment Phase of EMDR. It is possible to integrate Mapping and Graphing techniques (included in section 11 of this manual) during this phase of the EMDR protocol.

18. The therapist identifies general treatment goals with measurable behavioral objectives and completes the treatment plan form. For example, *"I know my child will have completed therapy when he/she has a 50% increase in successful school attendance."*

19. The therapist explains the Child/Adolescent Symptom Monitoring Form for use between sessions and gives the parent a copy of the Child/Adolescent Symptom Monitoring Form for parent use.

20. The therapist reviews treatment goals with the child and parent and answers any questions.

21. The therapist schedules the next appointment.

22. The therapist escorts the child and parent to the waiting room/exit.

Therapist Script for Client History and Treatment Planning

After interviewing the parent, bring the child into the session and utilize the following script when interviewing the child. *"What did your mom/dad/caretaker tell you about why you came here today?"* If the child does not respond, then the therapist continues with the following. *"Your mom/dad/caretaker told me that you had some worries, thoughts or feelings that are bothering you."* If no response from the child, the therapist offers some symptoms presented by the parent. For example, *"Your mom/dad/caretaker said you have bad dreams."* Continue: *"I'm wondering if there are other things that are bothering you that your mom/dad/parents/caretaker doesn't know about that we should talk about today."* Based on the therapist's attunement with the child, the therapist first attempts to have the child verbalize the target, but the child may need alternative options. *"If you want to, we can draw a picture or put all those things that are bothering you on my whiteboard so we don't miss any."* Allow the child to select the therapeutic tool to use in identifying targets for desensitization. The therapist can use sand tray, toys, or other activities to engage the child in identifying targets.

Intake Form for Child/Adolescent Psychotherapy

Child's name: _____ DOB/Age: _____ / _____

Child primarily lives with: ___ Both parents ___ Mother ___ Father ___ Other _____

Mother's name: _____ DOB: _____

Address: _____

Phone: (C) _____ (H) _____

Employer: _____

Custody: _____

Please list others living in mother's home, ages, and relationship to child:

_____

_____

Father's name: _____ DOB: _____

Address: _____

Phone: (C) _____ (H) _____

Employer: _____

Custody: _____

Please list others living in father's home, ages, and relationship to child:

_____

_____

Step-parent's/Guardian's information: (If applicable) _____

Address: _____

Phone: (C) _____ (H) _____

Employer: _____

Who has legal guardianship of your child? _____

Please describe custody and the child's current living arrangements: _____

Is there any legal involvement with your child? Yes _____ No _____ If so, please describe: _____

_____

Please bring copies of any court orders that impact your child.
Who are your child's significant others living with your child? Please list their names, ages, relationships, grades, and jobs if applicable:

1. _____

2. _____

3. _____

4. _____

Who are your child's significant others *not* living with your child? Please list their names, ages, relationships, grades, and jobs if applicable:

1. _____

2. _____

3. _____

4. _____

Intake Form for Child/Adolescent Psychotherapy (Page 2 of 2)

Child's name: _____ DOB/Age: _____ / _____

School attending and grade level (if applicable): _____

Child's job and employer (if applicable): _____

Work phone: _____ Work days and hours: _____

How were you referred: _____

Reason(s) for seeking therapy: _____

What goals do you have for therapy? _____

Have you sought mental health treatment before for your child? ___ Yes ___ No

If so, when and with whom? _____
_____

Current medical doctor/Family physician: _____

Phone number: _____

Current medications (type and dosage): _____
_____

Has there been any history or suspicion of physical, sexual, or emotional abuse? (If so please explain)
_____
_____
_____

Have there been any suicide attempts? (If so, explain) _____
_____

In case of emergency, please notify:

Name: _____ Phone: _____ Relationship: _____

Insurance (The following questions are about the policy holder.)

Policyholder's name: _____ SSN: _____ DOB: _____

Address: _____ City: _____ State: _____

Zip: _____

Home phone: _____ Work phone: _____ Cell phone: _____

Insurance company: 1. (*Medical*) _____

2. (*Mental health*): _____

Authorization #: _____ Number of sessions authorized: _____ Co-pay: _____

Employer: _____

Job title: _____

If you are a dependent, what is your relationship to the policyholder: _____

By completing this form, my signature indicates that the information provided is truthful and accurate.

Form completed by: _____ Date: _____

Signature: _____

EMDR Client History and Treatment Planning Form

(This form is completed in addition to the clinician's standard intake form.)

1. What are the parent's current concerns and goals for treatment? *("I know my child will have been successful in treatment when_____.")*

_____

_____

_____

_____

_____

_____

_____

_____

_____

2. Themes: (What themes are presented by child/parent related to responsibility, safety, control/choice?)

_____

_____

_____

_____

_____

_____

_____

_____

_____

_____

3. Symptom Assessment: (Does child/parent have any indication as to precursor of symptoms? How long have symptoms been present? Are there any times when symptom(s) are not present?)

_____

_____

_____

_____

_____

_____

_____

_____

4. Identify traumatic experiences as reported by parent only. The therapist asks the child to wait in play-room while interviewing the parent regarding targets. (What is the worst trauma experienced by the child per parent report? Assess for currently activated traumas including traumas/triggers most closely related to current distress or symptoms. Note any additional traumatic experiences spontaneously reported by the child. List triggers, that is, people, places, things, and so on that activate traumatic memories, cause distress or symptoms, or lead to avoidance.)

_____

_____

_____

_____

_____

_____

_____

_____

_____

_____

_____

_____

_____

5. Identify traumatic experiences as reported by the child. (The therapist asks the child to rejoin the session and interviews the child per the target identification script. The child may not identify any of the responses that the parent has identified.) The therapist also completes assessment tools (for a child 8 years or older) during this process. (The parent is asked to wait in the waiting room and complete the assessment tools if child is comfortable with the parent leaving.)

_____

_____

_____

_____

_____

_____

_____

_____

_____

_____

_____

_____

_____

6. Identify mastery experiences presented by the child. ("Tell me something that you are proud of that you have done. Tell me a time when you felt really good about yourself.")

_____

_____

_____

_____

_____

_____

_____

_____

_____

_____

_____

Notes:

_____

_____

_____

_____

_____

_____

_____

_____

_____

_____

_____

_____

_____

Clinician's name: _____ Date: _____

Clinician's signature: _____

Child Interview Questions

Child's name: _____ Date: _____

These questions are used to gather information from the child and build rapport in the therapeutic relationship. These questions can be used any time during the intake process. Any of the child's answers can be possible resources or targets for treatment.

1. Do you go to school? What school do you go to?

2. What's your teacher's name?

3. What is your favorite subject in school besides recess and lunch? (This usually gets a giggle from the child.)

4. If you had three wishes, what would they be?

5. What's your favorite color?

6. If you ruled the world, what would be two things you would change right away?

7. What's your favorite television program?

8. What makes you laugh?

9. What's your favorite sport or activity?

10. Tell me something that makes you sad.

11. What's your favorite animal?

12. Who lives at your house? (Explore people and pets.)

13. Who is your favorite superhero/heroine? (Possible resource)

14. Ask children about their bedroom. Who shares your room? Who decorated your room? What's your favorite thing in your room? (This question gets at information about the child's position in the family. Who makes decisions in the family? Is the child allowed to make decisions about their own room or did a parent decorate the room and did the child have any input?)

Child Interview Questions (Page 2 of 2)

Child's name: _____ Date: _____

1. What's your favorite movie? What's your favorite video game?

2. What do you do when you get really upset? Do you go to your room? Do you ride your bike or play video games or watch television?

3. Do you like to listen to music? What songs do you like the most? Do you ever listen to music when you're happy or upset?

4. Tell me something that is annoying to you. (If the child is someone who is bothered by tags, etc., this question may be more expansive.)

5. Who do you talk to when you're upset?

6. Who are your best buddies? What do you guys like to do together?

7. What do you do at recess?

8. Do you ever have headaches or stomach aches?

Therapist's notes:

_____

_____

_____

_____

_____

_____

_____

_____

_____

_____

_____

_____

_____

_____

Therapist's signature: _____ Date: _____

Consent for Treatment of Minor/Child Assent Form

Consent for Treatment of Minor

This is an authorization for _____ (therapist name) to provide treatment and/or diagnostic services to my child/adolescent, _____ (name). By signing this Consent for Treatment, I certify that I legally have custody or joint custody of my son or daughter and, thus, can legally consent for treatment of my child.

_____   _____

Parent/Guardian Signature   Date

Child Assent Form

I understand that my parent or guardian may consent for my treatment; however, I have also been asked to give my assent for my own treatment. By signing below, I realize that the therapist listed above has elicited my own assent for treatment.

_____   _____

Child's name   Birth date

_____   _____

Sign your name here   Witness

Treatment Plan

Client name: _____ Date: _____

Client ID #: _____ Therapist: _____

Current Behavioral Functioning Summary:

DSM-IV Diagnosis	Axis I:		
	Axis II:		
	Axis III:		
	Axis IV:	____ primary support	____ educational
		____ housing	____ social environment
		____ occupational	____ economic
		____ legal	____ access to health care
	Axis V:	____ current score	
		____ highest score past year	
		____ lowest score past year	

Problem Statements	Goals/Objectives Client Is to Achieve	Target Date

Treatment Plan (Page 2 of 2)

Client name: _____

Date: _____

Client ID #: _____

Therapist: _____

Mode of treatment

[ ] Individual   [ ] Group   [ ] Parent/Child dyad

[ ] Assessment

[ ] Court-ordered   [ ] Family   [ ] Supervised visit

Frequency of Treatment _____

_____

Treatment Methodology

[ ] Anger Management   [ ] Conflict Resolution

[ ] Problem-Solving Skills   [ ] Art Therapy

[ ] Desensitization   [ ] Psychoeducational

[ ] Assertiveness Training   [ ] Feeling Identification

[ ] Relaxation/Stress Mgmt   [ ] Assessment

[ ] Grief Work   [ ] Safety Planning

[ ] Behavior Modification   [ ] Insight Oriented

[ ] Sand Tray   [ ] Play Therapy

[ ] Bonding/Attachment   [ ] Music Therapy

[ ] Trauma Focused   [ ] EMDR

[ ] Parent Training   [ ] Communication Skills

Other _____

_____   _____

Client/Legal guardian signature   Date

_____   _____

Therapist signature   Date

Date of review   _____

(6 months from client signature)

Child/Adolescent Symptom Monitoring Form

Date: _____ Child's Name: _____

Parent Completing Form: _____

Therapist: _____

Symptoms	Day by Day (Following Therapy)						
	Day 1	*Day 2*	*Day 3*	*Day 4*	*Day 5*	*Day 6*	*Day 7*
Stomach aches							
Diarrhea/Constipation							
Sleep Disturbance							
Behavioral Problems							
Tantrums/Acting Out							
Crying							
Avoidance Behaviors							
Agitation							
Urination/Bowel Problems							
Refusal Behavior							
Anxiety							
Change in eating habits							
Headaches							

Note: 1 = minimal, 2 = moderate, 3 = severe

Other symptoms possibly related to treatment:

Symptoms	Day by Day						
	Day 1	*Day 2*	*Day 3*	*Day 4*	*Day 5*	*Day 6*	*Day 7*

Note: 1 = minimal, 2 = moderate, 3 = severe

Additional Comments/Concerns:

_____

_____

_____

_____

_____

_____

_____

_____

_____

Please complete this form and bring it to your child's next session. Thank you!

EMDR Progress Note

(This progress note is utilized after intake when Client History and Treatment Planning is completed, for initial or subsequent sessions starting with the Preparation Phase of EMDR.)

Review the developments since the last session (affective, somatic, cognitive, behavioral, imagery, symptoms, environmental changes. Therapist makes notes of any new concerns or changes in the child's life).

_____

_____

_____

Preparation: (What skills/resources does the child have and what skills/resources does the child need to continue with the EMDR protocol?)

_____

_____

_____

_____

Following the Targeting Sequence Identified as part of Client History and Treatment Planning or if the therapist previously started Assessment and Desensitization of targets.

_____

_____

_____

_____

_____

SUD on previous session's target (0–10) (Note particular type of measurement used by the child.):

_____

_____

_____

VoC on previous session's positive cognition (1–7) (Note particular type of measurement used by the child.):

_____

_____

_____

_____

Body scan on previous session's target (Note location of any negative or positive body sensations reported.)

_____

_____

_____
_____
_____

Target Identification

Memory/Target for current session (target from previous session/new target):

_____
_____
_____
_____

Assessment

Picture:

_____
_____
_____
_____
_____

Negative cognition:

_____
_____
_____
_____
_____

Desired positive cognition:

_____
_____
_____
_____

VoC: 1   2   3   4   5   6   7

    (completely false)   (completely true)

Client: _____ Therapist:_____

Date: _____ Visit: _____

18

Emotions

_____

_____

SUD

0   1   2   3   4   5   6   7   8   9   10

Neutral, no disturbance   Worst disturbance

_____

_____

Body sensations (location and description)

_____

_____

_____

Resources

Resources used:

_____

_____

_____

Closure

SUD at end of session (0–10):

_____

_____

VoC (if applicable) at end of session (1–7):

_____

_____

Body scan (Note location of any negative or positive body scan reported.)

_____

_____

Completed session: ❑ YES   ❑ NO

_____

_____

Closure exercise used (i.e. Safe/Calm Place, Relaxation Exercise, Containers):

_____

_____

Additional notes on back? ❑ YES   ❑ NO

_____

_____

_____

_____

_____

_____

_____

_____

_____   _____

Therapist's Signature   Date

Section 2

Preparation Phase

This section relates to chapter 4 of the book, *EMDR and the Art of Psychotherapy With Children.*

Introduction to EMDR, Mechanics of EMDR, Stop Signal, Metaphor, Safe/Calm Place, and Containers

The Preparation Phase establishes the foundation for continuing with the procedural steps of EMDR. This phase captures multiple areas that are the foundation for therapy, including establishing a therapeutic relationship and engaging the client in the therapeutic process, explaining EMDR, acquiring informed consent for EMDR treatment as necessary, assessing the client's resources and skills, assessing the client's home environment, determining what individuals will need to be included in the psychotherapy, and finally teaching the mechanics of EMDR. (See chapter 4 in *EMDR and the Art of Psychotherapy With Children.*)

In this section, additional instructions to the therapist are included with each EMDR mechanics protocol, including Stop Signal, Metaphor, Safe/Calm Place, and Container. Each protocol is designed to stand alone in order that the therapist can implement the protocol to create the foundation for proceeding with EMDR treatment.

This section offers guidance to the therapist for changing EMDR language into developmentally fitted sessions for children. Teaching the child the mechanics of EMDR creates the groundwork for treatment with multiple goals, including additional assessment of the child's ability to participate in treatment, understanding how the child processes, attunement to the child, and how the child deals with emotional intensity, as well as the child's skills at emotional regulation.

Session Protocol for the Preparation Phase

1. The therapist greets the child and parent in the waiting room and escorts them to the therapist's office.

2. The therapist reviews the first session and answers any questions from the child and parent. The therapist assesses general functioning since the initial session. The therapist reviews current status of any symptoms identified in the initial session and explores any new symptoms. *"Has anything changed since our last session?"* The therapist reviews any symptoms identified on the Child/Adolescent Symptom Monitoring Form and notes changes.

3. The therapist presents the therapeutic rationale for EMDR (Introduction to EMDR Treatment for Children, page 23).

4. The therapist explains the mechanics of EMDR and explores various forms of bilateral stimulation (BLS) with the child (Script for Mechanics, page 24).

5. The therapist teaches Stop Signal (Stop Signal Script, page 25).

6. The therapist teaches Metaphor (Metaphor Script, page 26).

7. The therapist provides an explanation/rationale for the Safe/Calm Place Exercise to the child and parent (Safe/Calm Place Script, page 28). The therapist completes Safe/Calm Place Worksheet (Safe/Calm Place Worksheet, page 29).

8. The therapist instructs the parent to remind the child to practice on a daily basis to connect with the imaginal Safe/Calm Place.

9. The therapist teaches the Container Exercise (Container Exercise Script, page 31).

10. The therapist reviews the session with the child and parent and answers questions as needed.

11. The therapist reminds the child and parent to practice Safe/Calm Place for enhancement between sessions.

12. The therapist reviews the Container Exercise and explains how the child can use containers between sessions.

13. The therapist schedules the next session and escorts the child and parent to the waiting room.

Introduction to EMDR Treatment for Children

Instructions to the Therapist for EMDR Treatment for Children

Explaining EMDR to parents is a straightforward process of educating parents about EMDR, what it is, how it works mechanically, and what it can do for their child. The therapist can reference the research on brain functioning and the mind/body connection. The therapist can also explain that the child's behavior and symptoms may be the brain's and body's adaptive response to what has happened. Even though there is no longer trauma, the child is locked in a pattern of responding to anything that looks, sounds, smells, or feels like the original experience as if it is the actual experience. The therapist can also explain trauma to the parent using a broad definition and place emphasis on how his or her child will reprocess and integrate frightening, hurtful, or traumatic experiences.

Script for EMDR Treatment, Mechanics, and Bilateral Stimulation (BLS) for Children

"I want to show you something we call EMDR and see how it works for you." The therapist will utilize the language unique to the individual child.

"When we do the EMDR we use these tools. We can use all kinds of things for EMDR so let's find out which one works best for you." The therapist starts with eye movements and then moves to other types of bilateral stimulations as appropriate for the individual child.

"I want to show you this thing that I have." The therapist brings out the EMDR NeuroTek machine with buzzies. *"This thing tickles a little when you hold it in your Hands. Do you want to try?"* The therapist teaches the child how to use the NeuroTek and allows the child to experiment.

The therapist will assess the child's response to the machine. If the child is comfortable, the therapist continues. If the child appears uncomfortable with buzzies, then the therapist explores other types of BLS with the child. The therapist then will demonstrate audio BLS with the NeuroTek machine.

"It doesn't seem like you like the buzzies. I want to see if maybe you'd like to hear the sounds this machine can make instead?" The therapist demonstrates audio BLS and allows the child to experiment. If the child is comfortable with audio BLS, continue. Once the child is comfortable with some type of BLS, continue explaining EMDR.

"With the _____ (BLS) we're gonna have you think about that _____ (Target) and just see how that works for you."

"Do you have any questions about how this EMDR thing works?" If the child has questions, the therapist responds to the questions. Otherwise, the therapist continues with treatment protocol.

Teaching Children to Use the Stop Signal With EMDR

Instructions to the Therapist for Teaching Children the Stop Signal

Teaching the child a signal to stop or take a break from the processing/desensitization gives the child a sense of safety and control over the process.

Script for Teaching Children the Stop Signal

"Remember when we talked about using _____ (BLS)? Well, I want you to know that you can raise your hand and tell me that you need to stop or take a break. Let's practice what you would do if you wanted to tell me to take a break." Follow the child's lead. The therapist may need to demonstrate raising the hand like a stop signal. After the child has identified a stop signal the therapist will then repeat, *"So I will know you want to take a break or stop if you do/say _____."*

Metaphor for EMDR

Instructions to the Therapist for Teaching the Child the Metaphor

The purpose of the metaphor is to give the client a sense of distance from the intensity of the affect the client may experience during desensitization with EMDR. In addition, the metaphor is significant to processing because it conveys a sense of movement through the intense affect, which helps prevent the child from being overwhelmed by the potency of the emotion.

Script for Teaching the Child the Metaphor

"It's kinda good to have a way to help you feel like you can handle your thoughts and feelings so you can just notice it like stuff going by like a train where you just watch stuff going by the window." The train metaphor may not be in the child's realm of experience.

Other more current metaphors to try are:

"Imagine that you are in a car or bus and you are just watching out the window at the bad thing passing by."

"Imagine that you're in a plane and can change your seat or look out the window."

Introduction to Safe/Calm Place

Instructions to the Therapist for Teaching Safe/Calm Place to the Child

The client is taught a safe/calm place to utilize as a tool for affect management. When clients can't locate a safe/calm place, consider that diagnostic and that the client is in need of additional resources including Resource Development and Installation (RDI) before continuing with desensitization. The therapist may need to use words other than *safe* such as *calm* or *happy* or other language unique to the individual child.

If the therapist continues with Safe/Calm Place Protocol, the therapist uses a maximum of two to four saccades of BLS at a slow speed in order not to bridge into trauma memories. If the child's identified safe place becomes unsafe, then the therapist asks the child, *"Can we make this safe place feel safe again or do we need to choose a different safe place?"*

Script for Teaching Safe/Calm Place to the Child

"OK, so I want to do something that's called Safe/Calm Place. We can use Safe/Calm Place at the end of sessions or between sessions. I want you to learn how to use Safe/ Calm Place, so we're going to practice it."

Step 1: Picture (Image): *"Can you think about a real place, or imaginary place that makes you feel safe/calm/relaxed or happy? What place makes you feel this way the most? Do you have a picture of it?"* (If appropriate, the therapist allows the child to draw a picture of the image.)

Step 2: Emotions and sensations. *"Think about that safe/comfortable/relaxed place. What feeling do you have?"* (Therapist pauses; if the child does not respond, therapist provides examples of feelings to educate child.) *"Do you feel relaxed, comfortable, safe, happy, excited? Where do you feel that ____ feeling in your body?"* (Therapist pauses, and if the child appears confused, therapist provides examples.) *"Well, some kids feel it in their heads, some people feel it in their tummy, some feel it in their heart. Where do you feel it? Can you touch it?"*

Step 3: Enhancement: The therapist then says, *"Think about that ____ picture, and that ____ feeling, and where you feel it in your body, and let's turn on ___ [BLS] for a few seconds."* Stop BLS and say, *"Tell me what happened now?"* (If the child feels better, the therapist should do several more sets of BLS. If the child's positive emotions do not intensify, the therapist can try alternative BLS until the child reports improvement.)

Step 4: Cue word(s): *"If we could pick one word that would help to remind me how you feel right now, what word would that be? (Pause for response.) Ok, so when I say ____, what do you notice?"* (Add a set of BLS.)

Step 5: Self-cuing: *"Now I want you to say the word ____ and when you say it notice what you're feeling."*

Step 6: Cuing with disturbance: *"Now let's practice with your word. I want you to think about one little tiny thing that bothers you just a little bit and notice where you feel that in your body."* (No BLS used at this point.)

Step 7: Self-cuing with disturbance: The therapist then asks the client to bring up a disturbing thought once again and to practice the Safe/Calm Place exercise, this time without the therapist's assistance, to its relaxing conclusion.

Step 8: Homework: Encourage the client to practice Safe/Calm Place Exercise and the word for cuing the safe/calm place.

Form for Safe/Calm Place:

Safe/Calm Place Worksheet

Image: _____

_____

_____

_____

_____

_____

Positive emotions: _____

_____

_____

_____

_____

_____

Physical sensations (location and description): _____

_____

_____

_____

_____

_____

_____

_____

Cue word(s): _____

_____

_____

_____

_____

_____

Minor disturbance for cuing/self-cuing practice: _____

_____

_____

_____

_____

Safe/Calm Place Protocol Abbreviated Instructions Form

Step 1: Describe image.

Step 2: Describe emotions and positive sensations (including location).

Step 3: Enhance imagery and affect with soothing tones.

Step 4: Introduce short sets of BLS (2–4 saccades).

   If positive outcome, continue with several more short sets.

   If minimal or neutral outcome, try alternative direction of BLS.

   If intrusions or negative response, explore solutions (e.g., containment of negative material, add more protective features to Safe/Calm Place) or switch to a different Safe/Calm Place or comforting resource image.

Step 5: Identify cue word(s). Guide the child in holding cue word(s) and Safe/Calm Place together as several sets of BLS are added.

Step 6: Have the child practice self-cuing, focusing on image and word(s) without BLS.

Step 7: Have the child bring up a minor disturbance. The therapist cues the Safe/Calm Place.

Step 8: Have the child bring up a minor disturbance. The child cues the Safe/Calm Place.

Containers for Children

Instructions to the Therapist for Teaching Containers for Children

Containers are used to assist children to close incomplete sessions and as another resource for affect management, especially between sessions. Containers can also be used to store new skills a child has learned for use in the future when they encounter situations that have previously been problematic. Using containers too early can provide the child with a technique to avoid reprocessing. It is important to teach the child that containers are temporary, but eventually the goal is to empty the container.

Script for Containers for Children

"Sometimes we have thoughts or feelings that get in our way at school or at home. Do you ever have thoughts or feeling like that? Well, I want you to know that if we need to we can put those thoughts or feelings in a container like a box or something really strong so that they can't get out. What do you think we could use to hold those thoughts or feelings?" Children may need to be taught examples. *"I want you to be able to put all of those thoughts or feelings, or what we worked on today, in that container. Sometimes we need different containers for different thoughts or feelings. Sometimes, I like to draw pictures of my _____ (container) and make sure it's strong enough to hold everything that I need it to hold. Would you like to draw a picture with me?"* After the child identifies a container, proceed by asking the child, *"OK, so we drew a picture* (note how the child identified the container) *of it, so now let's imagine that everything we worked on today is put in the container and we lock it away/seal it away until we get together again and can take it out to work on it again. When we get together we will work to empty your container so there's always room for new stuff if you need it. If you start thinking about things that bother you that are too hard to handle or they seem to come out before our next session, you can just imagine putting them into the container and giving it to me or making sure that I have it."*

Section 3

Assessment Phase

This section relates to chapter 5 of the book *EMDR, and the Art of Psychotherapy With Children.*

Instructions to the Therapist for the Assessment Phase

This chapter describes the procedural steps of the Assessment Phase of the EMDR protocol (Shapiro, 2001) with detailed explanations of the techniques and skills necessary for successfully steering a child through this phase, which are included in chapter 5 of the book *EMDR and the Art of Psychotherapy With Children.*

What is important for the therapist to recognize is that eliciting the procedural steps for the Assessment Phase is impacted by the child's level of development, and scripts for the procedural steps need to be adjusted into child language.

In order to help the therapist in the actual treatment process, we have included instructions to the therapist with scripts for each of the procedural steps of the Assessment Phase. At the end of the section we have then included one complete script for the procedural steps of the Assessment Phase to be used once the therapist feels comfortable eliciting the procedural steps.

This section starts with Target Identification, which is a continuation of what began during the Client History and Treatment Planning Phase. At this juncture, the therapist is asking the child to choose the target before proceeding with the procedural steps. The therapist should already have some idea of what the child may choose, given previous target identification procedures such as Mapping and Graphing. (See Section 11.)

Once the target has been selected, the therapist continues with Image, Negative and Positive Cognition, VoC, Emotion, SUD, and Body Sensation. We have artificially separated each procedural step for learning, with the understanding that eventually the therapist will use the complete script for the Assessment Phase, once the therapist becomes more familiar and comfortable with this phase of the protocol.

Session Protocol for the Assessment Phase

1. The therapist greets the child and parent in the waiting room and escorts them to the therapist's office.

2. The therapist reviews the previous session and answers any questions from the child and parent.

3. The therapist assesses general functioning since the previous session. The therapist reviews the current status of any symptoms identified in previous sessions and explores any new symptoms. *"Has anything changed since our last session?"* The therapist reviews any notations from the parent on the Child/Adolescent Symptom Monitoring Form.

4. If the therapist determines that the child does not have adequate resources, the therapist uses clinical judgment as to the child's need for Resource Development Installation. (See RDI Protocol in Section 10 of this manual.) If the therapist determines that the child has adequate resources, the therapist continues with the protocol as follows.

5. The therapist identifies targets for EMDR trauma processing with the child and parent. The therapist identifies traumatic memories/targets related to the experiences identified in numbers 4 and 5 in the EMDR Client History/ Treatment Planning Form on page 9 of this manual.

6. The therapist reviews the list of designated EMDR targets and the proposed treatment plan with the client and reviews the targeting sequence.

7. The therapist provides an explanation of the procedural steps in EMDR and specific instructions to the child about his/her participation in the treatment. (Procedural steps outline.)

8. Re-establish the setting in the office to provide for child comfort for EMDR processing. Review (BLS) as utilized in Safe/Calm Place and RDI exercises.

9. Begin EMDR (Assessment, Desensitization, Installation, Body Scan, Closure) based on the treatment plan target sequence. (The therapist uses the protocol labeled "Therapist Instructions/Script for Phases 3–4 of EMDR" starting on page 33 of this manual.) Complete as much work as time and circumstances allow, leaving adequate time for closure and debriefing.

10. If the session is incomplete, remind the client of the Container Exercise and other relaxation techniques to prepare the child for ending the session.

11. The therapist instructs the parent to remind the child to practice the Safe/ Calm Place Exercise between sessions in order to strengthen the Safe/Calm Place.

12. The therapist instructs the parent and child to practice the Container Exercise as necessary between sessions.

13. The therapist provides an additional Child/Adolescent Symptom Monitoring Form to parent.

14. The therapist schedules the next appointment and escorts the child and parent to the waiting room/exit.

15. The therapist completes the EMDR Progress Note.

Script for Reviewing the Previous Session

After bringing the child and parent into the office together, check in to get updates since the last session. Ask both the child and parents, *"Is there anything that has come up since our last session together?"* Ask to review the Child/Adolescent Symptom Monitoring Form to review symptoms including any changes of previously identified symptoms or new symptoms. After checking in with the child and parents, it is the therapist's decision whether or not to continue with the parent in the session. You may choose to ask the parent to wait in the waiting room while working with the child, or some therapists keep the parent in the office while working with the child. This decision is based on the therapist's preference for clinical practice.

The session now focuses on the child. The therapist begins by reviewing the mechanics of EMDR that were taught to the child in the previous sessions.

Review stop signal: *"If at any time you feel you want to stop, remember that you told me that you would do _____"* [stop signal previously identified].

Review and check Safe/Calm Place and resource images: Briefly review the safe/calm place and resource images established in earlier sessions.

"Remember that safe place that we talked about before?" (Therapist names the Safe/Calm Place and offers descriptive cues.) *"We can use that safe place when we are talking about what you remember, if you need to. I also want to make sure you remember what you told me about _____."* (Therapist describes resource images and associated feelings, qualities, or capacities if needed.) Optional: *"Do any of these _____* [resources] *feel like they could really help us right now? Do you think there are any people, pets, or objects that you would want sitting with you who could help you feel better when we talk about that thing that happened?"*

The therapist can use the EMDR Progress Note Form again here.

Target Identification for Children

Instructions to the Therapist for Target Identification

The therapist decides, in collaboration with the child and parent, what to target based on symptom presentation and on the list of traumatic experiences established during the Client History and Treatment Planning Process. Therapists can use Mapping and Graphing techniques included in section 11 of this manual for target identification.

It is important for therapists to recognize that often children's targets are more current. It is also notable that what the child identifies as the trauma may not be what the parent identifies as the trauma. We recommend that when choosing a target to reprocess, the therapist should select the target most associated with the current active symptoms the child is experiencing. *The child may have multiple traumas, but the trauma that is triggering the worst of the current symptoms for the child should be targeted first.* This can be determined during the history-taking portion of the first phase of EMDR. We encourage therapists to allow the child to guide the process and ask the child what target they want to start with in EMDR. This serves to empower the child and engage the child in treatment.

Then the therapist should proceed by asking the child, *"Can you remember a time when you felt like this before?"* This is still addressing the current target but tracing the channel to the past to see if there is an associated memory. Children frequently stay with the current target, which is fine. Frequently children will say, "No I don't remember another time," even if there was one. If they have no previous associated memory, target the current one.

When you choose the target connected to the worst of the current active symptoms you may also have a generalized desensitization effect on other traumas. A child may have a previous incident of molestation or physical abuse that may get completely reprocessed by targeting the current trigger or symptom. Thus, a generalization effect can occur with children unexpectedly.

The therapist can use drawing, clay, sand tray, and other techniques to elicit the worst part of the memory that is associated with the symptom or trauma. This requires that the therapist have patience and become attuned to the child, because the target and/or worst part of the memory may be expressed in nonverbal ways. As a last resort, if the therapist assesses that the child is completely unable to access the memory networks that are believed to be associated with the current symptoms, the therapist can request that the parent provide suggested targets along with possible negative and positive cognitions.

Once the therapist has determined that an appropriate target has been identified, the therapist can simply ask the child if the session can proceed with that target.

Script for Target Identification

"We have talked about things that worry or bother you before and, remember, we picked this one from your map, so how about we start with that one today?" Once the target has been chosen, the next step is to identify the picture or image that represents the worst part of the target.

Identifying Picture/Image

Instructions to the Therapist for Identifying Picture/Image

The goal for this section is to find a way of helping the child to express the worst part of the image from the target. The therapist can use art, sand tray, play therapy, or other techniques that are described in detail in chapter 5 of the book, *EMDR and the Art of Psychotherapy With Children*. Once the child has identified the image that represents the worst part, the therapist proceeds with eliciting the negative and positive cognition.

Script for Identifying Picture/Image

Most disturbing: *"What's the worst/yuckiest part of the incident?"* If the child identifies a picture or image, sound, smell, body sensation, continue with negative cognition.

If no picture: *"When you think about that thing, what happens now?"*

Eliciting Negative and Positive Cognitions

Instructions to the Therapist for Eliciting Negative and Positive Cognitions

We have changed the language to "what's the bad thought and what's the good thought?" Even little children can grasp that concept, but the negative cognition (NC) may be more trauma-specific. Also, the NC that the child identifies may not be what the parent thinks the NC is for the child. It is important that the NC resonates for the child. Depending on a child's development, the child may not always use "I" statements. The child may speak in third person, such as, "David hurt," with a positive cognition (PC) of "David feel better." These all relate to the child's current level of cognitive development or language acquisition. Sometimes the cognition is concrete, like "Jeff bad" versus "Jeff good." Or the child may use fantasy to express thoughts about himself or herself. Sometimes you get the PC first and then work backwards to get the NC. Just as with adults, the NC and the PC should resonate for the child. When it resonates, the child may tell you in a variety of ways; the child can make eye contact, say it, change his/her body language, change his/her play, or otherwise indicate it. (We have included a handout on NC and PC for kids.)

We have also included tips for eliciting negative and positive cognitions for children. Even though these tips may imply that the therapist is to eliminate some of the criteria for negative and positive cognitions, the intention is to keep the spirit of the NC/PC within Adaptive Information Processing theory based on the developmental mastery of the individual child.

To be more successful eliciting positive and negative cognitions with children, keep the following in mind:

- What parent(s) identify as traumatic is not necessarily what the child identifies.

- Self-referencing—Depending on the child's development the child may not always use "I" statements.

- Children tend to be concrete at times, and at other times may appear to be very obscure.

- Children are more likely to be trauma-specific.

- Older children may originally not be able to come up with an "I" statement but may come to it eventually if the therapist discusses their statements with the child.

- Sometimes you can work backwards by getting the positive thought first.

- NC and PC may first surface in pictures and play.

NC and PC may be single emotional words like sad vs. glad. If the child has verbalized an emotion, that can be the cognition, because developmentally the ability to verbalize a feeling indicates the child has moved beyond just experiencing the feeling into a cognitive process of verbalizing the feeling.

Children may express a negative cognition in the third person in order to protect themselves from the full impact of the cognition. In addition, younger children tend to use speech that is telegraphic such as "David hurt" and a positive cognition of "David feel better." The therapist can assist the child by eliciting negative and positive cognitions utilizing knowledge of the child's current live stressors. For instance, if we know that Katie has to go to the doctor, the therapist might say "Doctor scary" and then suggest that "Doctor fix Katie's owie."

In addition, children may provide very concrete NC and PC, like "Jeff bad" vs. "Jeff good." These concrete cognitions are often related to the child's current level of cognitive development and language acquisition. While some children present NC and PC in very concrete terms, other children may utilize fantasy to express their thoughts about themselves. For instance, 6-year-old Mollie may say, "I'm a witch" vs. "I'm a princess." The child's current media exposure can contribute to the child's expressions related to what he or she thinks about himself or herself.

Children tend to be more trauma-specific when identifying their NC and PC, such as, "I was scared of the dog" vs. "The dog can't get me anymore." For Melissa, being scared of the dog is related to having been unable to protect herself, while she may also be feeling unsafe in the environment in which she currently lives.

Children who struggle with verbalizing NCs and PCs can find greater capacity to express themselves through drawings, sand tray, and other expressive techniques. For instance, asking the child to create his or her worst world in one area of the sand tray while creating his or her best world on the other side may lead to identifying cognitions.

Ultimately, it is important to take the time to elicit negative and positive cognitions from children in order to be most effective with EMDR. As with adults, the negative and positive cognitions should resonate for the child. Children will often make eye contact, give verbal feedback, or change direction in their play behavior when the NC or PC fits. When the most appropriate NC and PC are identified for the child, the next phases of EMDR tend to be more valuable.

Script for Eliciting Negative and Positive Cognitions

Negative cognition (NC): *"When you think about that thing/picture, what words go with that?"* Or, you can say, *"What's the bad thought that goes with that,"* especially with younger children who may need education.

Positive cognition (PC): *"When you think about that thing/picture, what words would you rather say to yourself instead?"* Or you can say, *"What's the good thought that you want to tell yourself instead?"*

Tips for Eliciting the Touchstone Event

This is where some therapists may be confused about getting the Touchstone Event, which is the original incident that is believed to be at the root of the current symptoms. In the present, the symptom may manifest in a negative belief, a disturbing emotion, or an uncomfortable body sensation. These beliefs, emotions, or body sensations are clues to be used to track back to the original event with any age client. With children, the associative chaining that has brought the child from the disturbing event to the current symptom presentation may be the same event, because young children have shorter memory networks. During the Assessment Phase, there are different points when the therapist can use techniques to explore with the child the possible Touchstone Event. It is possible the Touchstone Event is a recent event, because children are more concrete and present-oriented. We recommend that therapists not assume that the child cannot identify an earlier incident, because with children it is much less likely that there is an earlier incident. This is where the Floatback Technique, Floatback Cognitive Interweave (See *EMDR and the Art of Psychotherapy With Children*), or Affect Scan can be used as is indicated to identify a Touchstone Event.

Kids' List of Cognitions

Bad Thoughts (NC)	Good Thoughts (PC)
I'm bad.	I'm good.
I'm in a fog.	I'm in a clear place/I'm in sunshine.
I'm going to blow.	I'm calm.
I'm going to explode.	I'm calm.
I'm hot.	I'm cool (as a cucumber).
I don't belong.	I do belong.
I'm stupid.	I'm smart.
I'm dumb.	I'm smart.
I'm sick.	I'm all better.
I can't do it.	I can do it.
I'm hurt.	I'm better.
I don't understand.	I do understand.
I can't get help.	I can get help.
I messed up.	I did the best I could.
I don't know nothing.	I do know.
I'm dying.	I'm alive.
I'm hungry.	I'm satisfied.
I'm not lovable.	I'm lovable.
I'm fat.	I'm just right.
I'm lost.	I found my way.
I almost drowned and I got very scared and that made me hold my breath.	I tell myself, you should be glad you could hold your breath that long.
I couldn't come out from under the water.	I'm glad I can swim.
I didn't get to go to the hospital with dad.	I get to go to the hospital with dad.
I'm not comfortable.	I am comfortable.
I am uncomfortable in my skin.	I fit in my skin.

Basic/Common Cognitions:

I'm not safe.	I'm safe now.
I can't protect myself.	I can protect myself.
I don't have control.	I do have control.
I can't trust.	I can trust.

Therapists can choose to organize NCs and PCs into categories of Safety, Responsibility, and Choice; however, often kids' cognitions are so concrete that it is difficult to determine the specific category in which the NC or PC falls.

This can be laminated and used for children who can read.

Measuring Validity of Cognition (VoC)

Instructions to the Therapist for Measuring the VoC

When measuring the Validity of Cognition (VoC), children often need simple instructions and a way to concretize the measurement. Given the child's development and the therapist's attunement to the child, the therapist can use different techniques described in the book, *EMDR and the Art of Psychotherapy With Children* to measure the VoC.

Script for Measuring VoC

"When you say those words_____ (repeat the PC), how true do those words feel right now, from 1, that means it's not true at all, to 7, that means it's really true?" (The therapist can use distance between the hands or other types of measures to which the child relates that are developmentally appropriate to demonstrate the validity of the cognition.)

Once the Validity of the Cognition has been measured, the therapist proceeds with having the child identify the emotion associated with the disturbing incident.

Identifying Emotions/Feelings

Instructions to the Therapist for Identifying Emotions/Feelings

Because the therapist has taught the child feeling identification and skills related to emotional literacy during the Preparation Phase, the therapist asks the child to identify a feeling associated with the incident.

Script for Identifying Emotions/Feelings

"When you bring up that picture (or incident) *and words* ____ (negative cognition), *what do you feel now?"* If the child needs further explanation, the therapist can use the feelings chart or some other type of educational tool to help the child identify emotion. Explore the emotion(s) that the child feels in the present.

Measuring Subjective Units of Disturbance (SUD)

Instructions to the Therapist for Measuring the SUD

Similar to the VoC, children may need a concrete manner to measure the Subjective Units of Disturbance. Again we refer the therapist to the book for in-depth skills in measuring the SUD.

Script for Measuring the SUD

"From 0–10, where 0 is it doesn't bother you at all to 10 where it bothers you a lot, how much does that thing bother you right now?" The therapist can use distance between hands or another type of measure to which the child relates.

Identifying the Location of Body Sensations

Instructions to the Therapist for Identifying the Location of Body Sensations

The therapist should refer to any mindfulness techniques taught during the Preparation Phase. It is often helpful for the therapist to actively demonstrate how to scan the body for the location of any body sensations. Again, advanced techniques for teaching children to identify body sensations are taught in the book.

Script for Identifying the Location of Body Sensations

"Where do you feel it in your body?" If the child is not initially able to answer, the therapist reminds the child of earlier training in mindfulness or teaches the child mindfulness of body sensations by pointing to body parts as the therapist says, *"Sometimes people feel it in their head, or their tummy, or their feet. Where do you feel it in your body?"*

Explaining Desensitization to the Child

Instructions to the Child Before Beginning Desensitization

"What we're gonna do is we're going to do the ____ [BLS] on that thing _____ [target] and I'm going to do to it for awhile and then I'm going to stop and tell you to blank it out and take a breath and then we'll talk a little about it. Sometimes things will change and sometimes they won't. There is no right or wrong answer. What you think or feel is exactly what I want to know and you can tell me anything."

Once the therapist has given the child these instructions, the therapist moves to the Desensitization Phase.

We have included a complete script for the Assessment Phase for therapists who have advanced to understanding the concepts and just need the script.

Script for Procedural Steps Outline of the Assessment Phase

The procedural steps of the Assessment Phase are included in one connected script for ease of use during session with child.

Review stop signal: *"If at any time you feel you want to stop, remember that you told me that you would do _____ (stop signal previously identified)."*

Review and check safe/calm place and resource images: Briefly review the Safe/Calm Place and resource images established in earlier sessions.

"Remember that safe place that we talked about before?" The therapist names the Safe/Calm Place and offers descriptive cues. *"We can use that safe place when we are talking about what you remember, if you need to. I also want to make sure you remember what you told me about _____."* The therapist describes the resource images and associated feelings, qualities, or capacities if needed. Optional: *"Do any of these _____ (resources) feel like they could really help us right now? Do you think there are any people, pets, or objects that you would want sitting with you who could help you feel better when we talk about that thing that happened?"*

Target Identification

"We have talked about things that worry or bother you before and, remember, we picked this one from your map, so how about we start with that one today?"

Picture

Most disturbing: *"What's the worst/yuckiest part of the picture?"*
If no picture: *"When you think about that thing, what happens now?"*

Cognitions

Negative cognitions: *"When you think about that thing/picture, what words go with that?"* Or, you can say, *"What's the bad thought that goes with that?"* especially with younger children who may need education.

Positive cognition: *"When you think about that thing/picture, what words would you rather say to yourself instead?"* Or you can say, *"What's the good thought that you want to tell yourself instead?*

Validity of Cognition

Validity of Cognition (VoC): *"When you say those words _____ (repeat PC), how true do those words feel right now, from 1, that means it's not true at all, to 7, that means it's really true?"* The therapist can use distance between the hands or other types of measures to which the child relates that are developmentally appropriate to demonstrate the Validity of the Cognition.

Emotions

Emotions/Feelings: *"When you bring up that picture* (or incident) *and words _____ (negative cognition), what do you feel now?"* If the child needs further explanation, the therapist can use the feelings chart or some other type of educational tool to help the child identify emotion. Explore the emotion(s) that the child feels in the present.

SUD

SUD: *"From 0–10, where 0 is it doesn't bother you at all to 10 it bothers you a lot, how much does that thing bother you right now?"* Therapist can use distance between the hands or another type of measure to which the child relates.

Body Sensation

Location of Body Sensation: *"Where do you feel it in your body?"* If the child is not initially able to answer, the therapist teaches the child mindfulness of body sensations by pointing to body parts as the therapist says, *"Sometimes people feel it in their head, or their tummy, or their feet. Where do you feel it in your body?"*

Instructions to the Child Before Beginning Desensitization

"What we're going to do is we're going to the _____ [BLS] on that thing _____ [target] and I'm going to do it for awhile and then I'm going to stop and tell you to blank it out and take a breath and then we'll talk a little about it. Sometimes things will change and sometimes they won't. There is no right or wrong answer. What you think or feel is exactly what I want to know and you can tell me anything."

Section 4

Desensitization Phase

This section relates to chapter 6 of the book, *EMDR and the Art of Psychotherapy With Children.*

Instructions to the Therapist for the Desensitization Phase

The goal of the Desensitization Phase is to reprocess the maladaptively stored memory and bring the incident to adaptive resolution. This is the phase that can be very short, especially with children, or can take a long time depending on the complexity of the associative chaining associated with the current symptom presentation.

For therapists, the Desensitization Phase can bring many challenges, including learning how to stay out of the way of the client's reprocessing, while also knowing when the client is stuck or looping and a cognitive interweave is indicated. It is also important for the therapist to be able to tolerate intense affect and be able to assist the client with a tolerable speed of reprocessing that does not overwhelm and shut down the client. The therapist also needs to know the techniques for under-accessing when the client is reporting that nothing is happening.

With child clients, the therapist may need to change types of bilateral stimulation more often to keep the child engaged. The therapist may also need to include more activity in working with children as they reprocess the memory through play therapy, art therapy, drawing, or other expressive psychotherapeutic tools.

It is the role of the therapist to be patient and diligent in attunement to the unique reprocessing of the individual child in order to bring the disturbance to a SUD of zero, making it possible to proceed to the Installation Phase of EMDR. A SUD of zero related to the original target is the ultimate goal of the Desensitization Phase, no matter how many maladaptively stored events the child presents during the session. Following the client's lead is the most important course of action during this phase.

Session Protocol for the Desensitization Phase

1. The therapist greets the child and parent in the waiting room and escorts them to the therapist's office.

2. The therapist reviews the previous session and answers any questions from the child and parent.

3. The therapist assesses general functioning since the previous session. The therapist reviews the current status of any symptoms identified in the previous session and explores any new symptoms. *"Has anything changed since our last session?"* Ask both the child and the parent. (Refer to the book for detailed instructions).

4. The therapist reviews any notations from the parent on the Child/Adolescent Symptom Monitoring Form.

5. At this juncture, the therapist will have structured the therapy sessions such that after these first four steps, the therapist will conduct the procedural steps of the Assessment Phase and move to the Desensitization Phase in one session. The goal is to allow time to have completed the procedural steps and begin bilateral stimulation to reprocess the target memory in one session. If this is the first time the therapist has proceeded with the Desensitization Phase with this client, go to step 10 below. If the therapist started reprocessing a memory in a previous session, and if the session was complete or incomplete, the therapist proceeds with number 6.

6. Re-evaluation—The therapist obtains feedback on experiences/observations since the last session. Ask the child to return to the target or incident from the previous session per the script. Check SUD and VoC on the previous target. Check for any unprocessed material from the previous session and probe for any new material that might have emerged.

7. If the child appears stable, the therapist proceeds with standard EMDR protocol. If the child appears unstable, the therapist continues with resource work. The therapist must discriminate between disturbance caused by the situation/trauma and that caused by internal instability. The former should be processed, while the latter should be improved through strengthening resources.

8. Re-establish the setting in the office to provide for child comfort for EMDR processing. Review BSL as utilized in Safe/Calm Place and RDI Exercises.

9. If the SUD rating on the previous week's target is greater than 0, continue to reprocess this target. If the VoC rating for the previous week's target is less than 7 (and does not appear to be ecologically valid), continue to reprocess this target. If the previous week's target appears to be resolved (SUD = 0, VOC = 7) and complete body scan, then move on to the next target on the treatment plan target list *or* move on to target current triggers associated with the memory addressed in the previous session.

10. Establish the EMDR target and begin EMDR (Assessment, Desensitization, Installation, Body Scan, Closure). Target old "activated" memories/material first. Proceed to focusing on current/recent triggers and future templates *only* after a specific old "activated" memory has been completely processed.

11. Complete as much work as time and circumstances allow, leaving adequate time for closure and debriefing.

12. The therapist schedules the next session and escorts the child and parent to the waiting room/exit.

13. The therapist completes the EMDR progress note form.

Script for Desensitization

"I'd like you to bring up that picture" [label and describe using client's word], *and the words* [repeat the negative cognition in client's words], *the _____ feeling, and notice where you are feeling it in your body and _____."* [Therapist uses whatever BLS has been previously identified.]

Begin the BLS. (You established the BLS method and speed during the introduction to EMDR.)

At least once or twice during each set of BLS, or when there is an apparent change, comment to the client: *"That's it. Good. That's it."* With children, the type of BLS may need to be changed often in order to assist the child in sustaining attention.

If the child appears to be too upset to continue reprocessing, it is helpful to reassure the child and to remind the child of the metaphor identified with the child prior to processing. *"It's normal for you to feel more as we start to work on this. Remember we said it's like _____ [metaphor] so just notice it. It's old stuff."* (Use this only if needed, if the child is upset.)

After a set of EM, instruct the child by saying: *"Take a deep breath."* It is often helpful if the therapist takes an exaggerated breath to model for the child, as the therapist makes the statements to the child.

Ask something like: *"What did you get now?"* Or, *"Tell me what you got?"* Or if the child needs coaching, *"What are you thinking, feeling, how does your body feel or what pictures are you seeing in your head?"*

After the child recounts his/her experience, say: *"Go with that,"* and do another set of BLS. (Do not repeat the child's words/statements.) As an optional phrasing you can say, *"Think about that."*

Again ask, *"What do you get now?"* If new negative material presents itself, continue down that channel with further sets of BLS.

Continue with sets of BLS until the child's report indicates that the child is at the end of a memory channel. At that point, the child may appear significantly calmer. No new disturbing material is emerging. Then return to the target. Ask: *"When you think about that thing we first talked about today, what happens now?"* (Remember that children may not show affect and may often process very quickly. So there may be no more disturbing material for the child to access or describe about the target memory.) After the child recounts his or her experience (children may verbalize or draw *or* otherwise demonstrate through play therapy what they have experienced), add a set of BLS.

If positive material is reported, add one or two sets of BLS to increase the strength of the positive associations before returning to the target. If you believe the child is at the end of a channel, that is, the material reported is neutral or positive, then ask: *"When you go back to that first thing we talked about today* [therapist references the picture, sand tray, or whatever was used by the child to identify the original target], *what do you get now?"* Whatever the child reports, add a set of BLS.

If no change occurs, check the SUD. Ask the child, *"When you think about that thing, from 0–10 where 0 means it doesn't bother you at all to 10 meaning it bothers you a lot, how much does that thing bother you right now?"* (The therapist can use one of the alternate ways of checking the SUD described in the Assessment Phase.)

If the SUD is greater than 0, continue with further sets of BLS, time permitting. If the SUD is 0, do another set of BLS to verify that no new material opens up. Then proceed to the installation of the PC. (*Remember:* Only proceed to Installation after you have returned to the target, added sets of BLS, no new material has emerged, and the SUD is 0.)

Section 5

Installation Phase

This section relates to chapter 7 of the book, *EMDR and the Art of Psychotherapy With Children.*

Instructions to the Therapist for Installation

The goal for the Installation Phase is to check the original positive cognition to see if it still fits or if another one fits better and then to install the positive cognition until the client reports a VoC of 7.

The therapist has the child hold the original memory together with the positive cognition and asks the child to measure the VoC. If the VoC is not 7, the therapist proceeds to strengthen the VoC by adding a set of BLS. Each time the therapist uses a set of BLS, the therapist checks the VoC. This can be very annoying to children as they quickly move to a VoC of 7 and don't want to keep answering the same question.

During the Installation Phase, the therapist continues to use the same type, speed, and frequency of BLS as used during Desensitization, because it is important that any unresolved data emerges.

Session Protocol for Installation

The Installation Phase often occurs during the session immediately following the Desensitization Phase, when the client has reprocessed the maladaptively stored memory and the SUD is a 0. Typically a session would not begin with Installation unless the previous session ended at the conclusion of Desensitization, or, if upon re-evaluation the memory has reprocessed between sessions and even though the SUD was not at 0 at the end of the previous session, upon re-evaluation in this new session the SUD is now 0. If the client reported the SUD as 0, the therapist would begin the session as follows.

1. The therapist greets the child and parent in the waiting room and escorts them to the therapist's office.

2. The therapist reviews the previous session and answers any questions from the child and parent.

3. The therapist assesses general functioning since the previous session. The therapist reviews the current status of any symptoms identified in the previous session and explores any new symptoms. *"Has anything changed since our last session?"* Ask both the child and the parent. (Refer to the book for detailed instructions.)

4. The therapist reviews any notations from the parent on the Child/Adolescent Symptom Monitoring Form.

5. Because the client has reported that the SUD is now a 0 due to spontaneous reprocessing between sessions, the therapist proceeds with the steps of Installation using the script included later in the section.

6. Typically the Installation Phase does not take much time, especially with children, and after the VoC has strengthened and installed and the client is reporting a VoC of 7, the therapist proceeds with the Body Scan.

7. If Installation occurs at the end of the session, the therapist proceeds with closure of an incomplete session. Complete as much work as time and circumstances allow, leaving adequate time for closure and debriefing.

8. The therapist schedules the next session and escorts the child and parent to the waiting room/exit.

9. The therapist completes the EMDR Progress Note Form.

Script for Installation

Installing the positive cognition is about linking the desired positive cognition with the original memory/incident or picture:

"Do the words _____ [repeat the positive cognition] *still seem right, or are there other positive words that would be better now?"*

"When you think about that thing we talked about at the beginning and you say those words _____ [repeat the PC], *how true do those words feel right now from 1, it's not true at all, to 7, it's really true?"*

"Now think about that event and say those words, _____," [repeat PC] *"and follow."* Then do a set of BLS.

Then check the VoC again. *"When you think about that thing we talked about at the beginning and you say those words* _____ [repeat the PC], *how true do those words feel right now from 1, it's not true at all, to 7, it's really true?"*

Continue doing sets of BLS as in step 2, as long as the material is becoming more adaptive. If child reports a 7, repeat step 3, again to strengthen and continue until it no longer strengthens. Then go on to the Body Scan.

If after several sets of BLS the child still reports a 6 or less, check appropriateness of the PC and address any blocking belief (if necessary) with additional reprocessing.

Section 6

Body Scan Phase

This section relates to chapter 7 of the book, *EMDR and the Art of Psychotherapy With Children*.

Instructions to the Therapist for Body Scan

The goal of the Body Scan Phase is to guide the child through the steps to achieve a clear body scan. The therapist asks the child to scan their body using the script that follows in this section. If any sensation is reported, do a set of BLS. If a discomfort is reported—reprocess until the discomfort fully subsides. Then do the Body Scan again to see if there are still any negative sensations. If a positive or comfortable sensation is reported, do BLS to strengthen the positive feeling. If a sensation of discomfort is reported, do BLS to strengthen the positive feeling. Once the child achieves a clear body scan, the therapist then guides the child through the development of a positive template for future action.

Session Protocol for Body Scan

The Body Scan Phase often occurs during the session immediately following the Installation Phase, when the client has achieved a VoC of 7. Typically a session would not begin with Body Scan Phase unless the previous session ended at the conclusion of the Installation Phase. Or, the session may begin with the Body Scan if upon re-evaluation at the beginning of a new session, the VoC has strengthened, and even though the VoC was not at a 7 at the end of the previous session, upon Re-evaluation during this new session the client reports that the VoC is now a 7. If the client reported the VoC as a 7, the therapist would begin the session as follows.

1. The therapist greets the child and parent in the waiting room and escorts them to the therapist's office.

2. The therapist reviews the previous session and answers any questions from the child and parent.

3. The therapist assesses general functioning since the previous session. The therapist reviews the current status of any symptoms identified in the previous session and explores any new symptoms. *"Has anything changed since our last session?"* Ask both the child and the parent. (Refer to the book for detailed instructions.)

4. The therapist reviews any notations from the parent on the Child/Adolescent Symptom Monitoring Form.

5. Because the client has reported a VoC of 7, the therapist proceeds with the Body Scan.

6. Typically the Body Scan Phase does not take much time, especially with children, and after the child reports a clear body scan, the therapist proceeds with closure.

7. If the Body Scan occurs at the end of the session and a clear body scan is not achieved, the therapist proceeds with closure of an incomplete session. Complete as much work as time and circumstances allow, leaving adequate time for closure and debriefing. If new material arises, the therapist continues following the associative chaining until it dissipates. If it is clear that a new target has emerged, the therapist must determine how much time is left in the session. The therapist may choose to add this new target to the map and return to target the incident later.

8. If there is time remaining in the session, the therapist proceeds with desensitizing whatever the client reports. Complete as much work as time and circumstances allow, leaving adequate time for closure and debriefing.

9. The therapist schedules the next session and escorts the child and parent to the waiting room/exit.

10. The therapist completes the EMDR Progress Note Form.

Script for Body Scan

"Close your eyes; concentrate on that thing you told me about and the words _____ [repeat the final positive cognition] *and notice your whole body from the top of your head to the bottom of your feet and tell me where you feel anything."* If the child reports any sensations, add a set of bilateral stimulation. Then ask the child again, *"What are you noticing now?"* What children report varies, and the therapist's goal is to continue asking the child about any body sensations and then reprocessing with BLS.

If the child reports a clear body scan, continue with the next phase of treatment. Sometimes children may link up to another memory, and then the therapist must make a decision about whether what the child is reporting is a new target, a new channel, or whether it can be reprocessed with bilateral stimulation. For a more detailed explanation, the reader is referred again to the book, *EMDR and the Art of Psychotherapy With Children.*

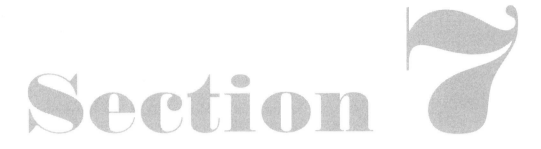

Section 7

| Closure Phase

This section relates to chapter 7 of the book, *EMDR and the Art of Psychotherapy With Children.*

Instructions to the Therapist for Closure

The Closure Phase of EMDR occurs anytime the therapist needs to close a session. The goal of the Closure Phase involves choosing an appropriate ending point for the session while assisting the client in debriefing and shutting down any disturbance that arose during the session. It is important to acknowledge the child for what he or she has accomplished and to leave the child well grounded before departing. Once the therapist has assisted the child in transitioning to a more comfortable state, the last goal of the Closure Phase is to prepare the child and parent for the time between sessions.

    We have included a general script for closing a session. We have then included as well directions for closing an incomplete session. An incomplete session is one in which a child's material is still unresolved, that is, they are still obviously upset or the SUD is above 1 and the VoC is less than 6.

Session Protocol for Closure

The Closure Phase often occurs during the session immediately following the Body Scan Phase, when the client has achieved a clear body scan. Typically a session would not begin with the Closure Phase. Closure is either at the end of a session or at the end of treatment. The scripts included here are for use at the end of a session. We have included two scripts. The first script is for when the target has been reprocessed and completed with a SUD of 0, VoC of 7, and a clear body scan. The second script is for when the target is not completed and the therapist is using closure for an incomplete target session.

Script for Closure

"Well we've done a lot of work today and you're awesome. Before I see you next time, you may think about stuff, so would you draw me a picture or write something down or tell your mom and dad if you have any thoughts, dreams, or feelings that you want to remember to tell me or would be good for me to know?" The therapist then reminds the child of resources for use between sessions. *"Remember to use your Safe/Calm Place, or your Containers, or talk to your parents if anything comes up that really bothers you a lot until we can talk next time. If you have any questions or if it bothers you a lot, you can have your mom or dad call me."*

Script for Closing Incomplete Sessions

Explain the reason for stopping and check on the child's state. *"We need to stop and clean up now because it's time to go. How're you doing after the thing we talked about today?"*

Give encouragement and support for the effort made. *"We worked hard today and you're awesome. How are you doing right now?"*

"Let's stop and do our Container and our Safe/Calm Place one more time before we go. Remember your Safe/Calm Place? I want you to think about that place. What do you see? What do you smell? What does it feel like to be there? Where do you notice it in your body?" The therapist uses the process to access Containers or the Safe/Calm Place.

Section 8

Reevaluation Phase

This section relates to chapter 8 of the book, *EMDR and the Art of Psychotherapy With Children.*

Instructions to the Therapist for Reevaluation

At the start of every session after EMDR has been introduced, the therapist assesses treatment progress and resolution of previously activated traumas. It is very important to do reevaluation with children, because children may not demonstrate much affect during desensitization. Reevaluation with children is the primary manner in which the therapist can assess the successful reprocessing of previously maladaptively stored information. The therapist can use the Mapping and Graphing to reevaluate the child's progress in treatment. As the ultimate goal of therapy, symptom reduction and alleviation is the evidence of treatment progress. It is through reevaluation that treatment outcome is measured.

Session Protocol for Reevaluation

1. It is important to note that typically at every session begins with Reevaluation.

2. The therapist greets the child and parent in the waiting room and escorts them to the therapist's office.

3. The therapist reviews the previous session and answers any questions from the child and parent.

4. The therapist assesses general functioning since the previous session. The therapist reviews the current status of any symptoms identified in the previous session and explores any new symptoms. *"Has anything changed since our last session?"* Ask both the child and the parent. (Refer to the book for detailed instructions.)

5. The therapist reviews any notations from the parent on the Child/Adolescent Symptom Monitoring Form.

6. The therapist reevaluates the previous target if all targets have not been reprocessed.

7. The therapist and client complete as much work as time and circumstances allow, leaving adequate time for closure and debriefing.

8. The therapist schedules the next session and escorts the child and parent to the waiting room/exit.

9. The therapist completes the EMDR Progress Note Form.

Script for Reevaluation

"Remember what we worked on last time, did you think about it at all? Was there anything that you wanted me to know since our last session?"

Ask the parent if there have been any changes since the last session (e.g., changes in symptoms, new behaviors, etc.).

The therapist reevaluates the degree of processing of the previous target to determine whether or not the target has been resolved (SUD = 0, VOC = 7). SUD of more than 0 or VoC of less than 7 is only acceptable if ecologically valid. The therapist reevaluates the SUD as the child focuses on the target from the previous session. If not a SUD of 0, what remains disturbing as the client holds the target in his or her awareness (image, cognition, emotion, sensation). *"When you go back to what we worked on last time, what do you get now?"* After the child answers, the therapist responds, *"When you think about that _____, (client's answer), how much does it bother you now?"* The therapist elicits SUD. The therapist continues by asking the child, *"And when you think about the thing we worked on and the thought _____* (the therapist repeats the client's PC from the previous session), *how true does that feel for you right now from 1, not true at all, to 7, totally true?"* The therapist can use hand distance or another measure previously utilized with the specific client.

The therapist continues with reprocessing with all targets associated with current symptoms until all the necessary targets have been reprocessed.

Final Desensitization/Trauma Processing Session

Instructions to the Therapist for Final Desensitization/Trauma Processing Session

As the treatment process nears completion, the therapist reviews the child's progress in treatment and begins to plan for discharging the child from care.

Session Protocol for Final Desensitization/Trauma Processing Session

1. The therapist greets the child and parent in the waiting room and escorts the child to the therapist's office.

2. The therapist reviews the previous session and answers any questions from the child and parent.

3. The therapist assesses general functioning since the previous session. The therapist reviews the current status of any symptoms identified in previous sessions and explores any new symptoms. *"Has anything changed since our last session?"* The therapist reviews any notations from the parent on the Child/Adolescent Symptom Monitoring forms.

4. The therapist reestablishes the setting in the office to provide for child comfort for EMDR processing and reviews BLS as utilized in Safe/Calm Place and RDI exercises.

5. The therapist notes any incomplete processing of targets to be completed in the session.

6. The therapist continues with EMDR treatment to complete any unresolved targets.

7. The therapist schedules the final session and reminds the client of goals for the final session, including posttest assessment. The therapist should leave adequate time for closure and good-byes during the session.

8. The therapist escorts the child and parent to the waiting room/exit.

9. The therapist completes EMDR Progress Note and Discharge Forms.

Reevaluation and Posttreatment Assessment

This session protocol is for the final sessions of treatment.

Session Protocol for Reevaluation and Posttreatment Assessment

1. The therapist greets the child and parent in the waiting room and escorts them to the therapist's office.

2. The therapist reviews the previous session and answers any questions from the child and parent.

3. Comprehensive reevaluation: the therapist assesses general functioning since the previous session. The therapist reviews treatment goals and assesses targets for any disturbance by taking a SUD for each target. This is conducted with both the child and parent in session.

4. If disturbance continues with any targets, the therapist notes the child's disturbance for processing.

5. The therapist explains to the child and parent that this is the final session and that treatment can continue in order to address any additional ongoing concerns that may arise in the future.

6. If treatment is completed, the therapist conducts the good-bye process.

7. If treatment is not completed, but the child and family have decided to end this episode of care, the therapist assists the child in planning for continued treatment or referral as appropriate.

8. The therapist administers posttest assessment tools with the parent.

9. The therapist reminds the child and parent to practice utilizing resources.

10. The therapist escorts the client and parents to the waiting room.

11. The therapist completes the EMDR Progress Note for discharge.

Form for EMDR Therapy Discharge/Discontinuation of Treatment

Child's Name: _____

Therapist's initials: _____ Date: _____

Number of intervention sessions completed: _____

Reason for ending treatment: _____

Completed protocol _____ Staff decision _____ Client decision _____

Treatment assessment (e.g., how child responded to EMDR; engagement with treatment; degree/kind of progress; explanation of early termination if applicable):

_____

_____

_____

_____

_____

_____

_____

_____

_____

_____

_____

_____

_____

_____

_____

_____

_____

_____

_____

_____

_____

_____

_____

_____

Therapist's signature_____ Date _____

Section 9

Cognitive Interweaves for Children

This section relates to chapter 10 of the book, *EMDR and the Art of Psychotherapy With Children.*

Instructions to the Therapist for Cognitive Interweaves for Children

A cognitive interweave is the elicitation of an adaptive perspective by the therapist that is offered when reprocessing is stuck, or when the child is looping, or when time is running out and it is necessary to expedite the session so that the child does not remain in a highly activated state. The cognitive interweaves can also be used to generalize positive associations beyond the original target, which is often difficult for children.

Cognitive interweaves are used to "jump-start" (Shapiro, 2001) the blocked processing when the previous approaches have not worked. The therapist introduces new material without relying on the child to provide it. It is a "light touch" to elicit certain information from the child's neuronetworks. The therapist initiates cognitive interweaves through questions or instructions that elicit thoughts, actions, or imagery. Cognitive interweaves should be used selectively so the child's own processing system can do the work, which provides full integration of information and is empowering to the child (Shapiro, 2001).

Cognitive interweaves for children fall mainly under the categories of safety, responsibility, choice, and empowerment. Usually cognitive interweaves are a question such as *"Are you safe now?"* (safety), *"Well whose job was it?"* (responsibility), or *"Are you making better choices now?"* (choices).

When utilizing a cognitive interweave, make sure it resonates for the child and stimulates his or her own internal resources. It is important for the therapist to be familiar with the child's culture and the current genre of that child's reality. What are the heroes in this child from movies, sports, school, or television that can be used for resourcing? The therapist uses one or more questions to guide the client to find an answer drawn from the child's own internal wisdom. The therapist may use Socratic questioning to access the child's own logic and to resume the child's own

69

natural processing. For example, *"If your friend was feeling the same way, what would you tell one of your friends?"*

Blocked processing basically means either the SUD are not going down or the child is overwhelmed by the intense emotion, which halts processing. The therapist may encounter the need for a cognitive interweave during any of the following.

Editing

During the Desensitization Phase, editing may be what is occurring when the child appears to have encountered blocked processing; however, the child may not have experienced blocked processing but instead may be editing. Editing occurs when the client reports his/her experience in general terms such as, "It's the same," or "Nothing," or "I'm numb." Children will say things like, "I feel nothing" instead of saying they feel numb. Ask the child in a respectful way to specifically describe everything they are getting. Or, ask the child to describe specifically what "nothing" is like. The therapist can also ask the child to describe numbness or nothingness and where he or she feels it in the body.

Looping

Looping is one form of blocked processing. Looping occurs when the child is saying the same thing in the same modality (e.g., cognitions, emotions, images, body sensations) at least two or three times, such as, "I'm bad" (cognition), "I'm scared, I'm scared" (emotion), "I see my mom standing on the stairs" (image), or "My stomach hurts" (body sensation). Looping is stuck processing. Looping is not the patient reporting sequences of trauma, which are really channels of association (Shapiro, 2001) or chaining. If the therapist believes the child is looping, the therapist should change speed, direction, or type of BLS. Or the therapist can ask the child to notice his or her body or notice where the body sensation is most pronounced. The therapist can also ask the child where they feel the negative cognition in their body. For example, if the negative cognition is "I'm bad," the therapist asks the child, *"Where do you feel that in your body?"* Find out what are the unspoken words, or have the child use movement, or press on the body where the sensation is in order to access an image or a thought or a memory. What this does is to find different aspects of the target.

Session Protocol for Cognitive Interweaves for Children

No session protocol is included for cognitive interweaves because cognitive interweaves are not delineated as a specific session but are used to assist with blocked processing and are integrated into other sessions' protocols as needed.

Example of Scripts for Cognitive Interweaves for Children

When a client is stuck at a SUD of 3 or less, the therapist can say to the child *"What would it take to get it to be a 0?"* (Or use an alternate phrase for the type of measurement the child has identified for measuring SUD). So if the child says, *"I need to feel safe,"* the therapist says, *"What would it take for you to feel safe?"* If the child responds with a realistic statement, the therapist then proceeds with further sets of BLS by directing the child to, *"Go with that."* If the child responds with an irrational or unrealistic statement, the therapist then goes through a series of questions to guide the child to an adaptive response. Once an adaptive response is elicited, then the therapist proceeds with further sets of BLS by saying, *"Go with that."*

Utilizing Cognitive Interweaves to Restart Processing

The following are types of cognitive interweave choices and examples of how to utilize them when appropriate:

New information: When the child has insufficient information, such as poor education, little experience in this area, or developmental capabilities that do not give the child enough information to process, then the therapist offers the following to assist the child with processing:

Child: I did something bad.

Therapist: Kids have to be taught how to get mad in the right way. It's a grown-up's job to teach kids this and show them how to do it. Nobody is born knowing how to do that. Did anyone teach you?

Child: No.

Therapist: Think about that.

The therapist continues with sets of 24 BLS. (Anywhere we have included the recommendation for "sets of 24 BLS," we are suggesting that the therapist needs to use whatever number of saccades he or she has been using during reprocessing.)

"I'm confused": The client has the information but the therapist uses another way of getting to that information.

Child: I could have stopped him.

Therapist: I'm confused. Are you saying a 40-pound 6-year-old can stop a 200-pound grown-up from hitting another grown-up?

"What if it were your best friend?": The therapist can use anyone the client feels lovingly protective of that would be an appropriate replacement in the incident.

Therapist: If this happened to your best friend what would you tell her?

Child: I'd tell her, "It's not your fault. Your mommy should've taken care of you."

The therapist continues with sets of 24 BLS.
Ask the child:

Therapist: What would it take to make that thing be only this up-setting? (using hands or other appropriate measures).

The therapist continues with sets of 24 BLS.
Change pictures, perspectives, and personal referent:

Therapist: What's the difference between then and now?

Child: I'm bigger.

Therapist: Think about that.

The therapist continues with sets of 24 BLS.

Metaphor/Analogy: Use to impact therapeutic lessons through stories, songs, poems, movies, TV shows, stories of other children's struggles.

Therapist:	Harry Potter didn't have his parents. How did he handle his loneliness at Hogwarts?
Child:	He talked to his friends and looked at their picture.
Therapist:	Think about that.

The therapist continues with sets of 24 BLS.

Or

When a client doesn't know how to handle another child's insults, use a story about the old rhyme, "I'm rubber and you're super-glue, whatever you say bounces off of me and sticks to you."

Therapist:	Think about that.

The therapist continues with sets of 24 BLS.

Socratic Method: Ask the client a series of questions that shapes the client's perspective. For example, if the client irrationally worries about his house burning down:

Therapist:	How old are you?
Child:	10.
Therapist:	That's pretty old.
Child:	Yeah.
Therapist:	Has your house ever caught fire before? (Make sure you know that the answer is no.)
Child:	No.
Therapist:	How old is your mother?
Child:	I don't know. Pretty old. Maybe 30-something.
Therapist:	Has her house or houses ever burned down? (Again, make sure you know the answer is no.)
Child:	No.
Therapist:	Think about that.

The therapist continues with sets of 24 BLS.

Or

Gifted kids often worry about nuclear war or getting diseases.

Therapist:	Less than 1% of children get deadly cancer. Did you know that?

Child: No.

Therapist: So if the weatherman told you there was less than a 1% chance of rain today, how likely do you think it would be that it would rain today? Would you bring your umbrella?

Child: No. I guess not.

Therapist: Think about that.

The therapist continues with sets of 24 BLS.
Designate appropriate responsibility:

Therapist: Who is supposed to take care of kids, grown-ups or kids?

Child: Grown-ups.

Therapist: Think about that.

The therapist continues with sets of 24 BLS.
Let's pretend: This helps the child think about other positive ways of change and can reduce fear.

Therapist: Let's pretend you could say anything you wanted and not worry about what would happen. What would you say?

Child: I hate you.

Therapist: Imagine saying that.

The therapist continues with sets of 24 BLS.
Or

Therapist: Let's pretend you were 10 feet taller, what would you do?

Child: I'd stomp on him and run away.

Therapist: Imagine doing that.

The therapist continues with sets of 24 BLS.
Or

Therapist: Do you know somebody either real or imaginary who could handle dealing with things without his/her parents being there?

Child: Like maybe Harry Potter?

Therapist: Think about that.

The therapist continues with sets of 24 BLS.
After the cognitive interweave is initiated do only 24 saccades of BLS to check in quickly in order to determine if the cognitive interweave worked to restart reprocessing. If the client rejects the cognitive interweave, be open to trying others.

Cognitive Interweaves for Current or Future Issues

Cognitive interweaves can also be used for stuck processing associated with current or future issues:

Assimilation: Helps to decrease strong emotions and give new information to develop positive future behaviors. Example: The client is still fearful even though the perpetrator is in jail.

Therapist: Can he hurt you now?

Client: No.

Therapist: Think about that.

The therapist continues with sets of 24 BLS.

Verbalizations and actions: The therapist can prompt the client with either verbalizations or actions to express or to practice future behaviors.

Therapist: What would you have liked to say to him?

Client: I'm gonna tell on you.

Therapist: Imagine that.

The therapist continues with sets of 24 BLS.

Therapist: Now say it out loud.

The therapist continues with sets of 24 BLS.

Resource Development and Installation for Children

This section relates to chapter 9 of the book, *EMDR and the Art of Psychotherapy With Children*. Resource Development and Installation (RDI) was created by Korn and Leeds (2002). The following section and protocols were developed from the work of Korn and Leeds.

Instructions to the Therapist for Resource Development and Installation for Children

The instructions for RDI with children need to be adapted in developmentally appropriate language. RDI should only be used when the child does not appear to have adequate tolerance to utilize EMDR.

Initially, the child is asked to focus on a problematic current life situation, or a blocking belief. The child is then asked to identify the qualities (or capacities, strengths, feelings, people, pets, or other resources) the child believes he or she needs in order to deal with this situation or belief. If the child identifies multiple qualities, the therapist asks the child to identify the quality that they think/feel would be most important to assist them with this specific situation. If necessary, this process is repeated for each of the qualities the child identifies.

The therapist uses knowledge of the child's history and current social and personal resources to help identify a mastery experience associated with this quality and with positive affect.

If such an experience cannot be recalled, the child is asked to remember someone else dealing effectively with this type of situation or someone who embodies the desired quality. The child can be asked to identify a person who is seen as a good coach, mentor, or support figure from their present or past. The person can be real or imaginary or can be from children's books, TV, games, videos, and so on.

BLS is utilized to install the resource, and if the resource experience is enhanced, the therapist continues with two to three saccades of BLS as long as positive feelings and associations get stronger. BLS is discontinued when the resource is optimally strengthened.

The bilateral stimulation is stopped if the child associates to negative material. In this case, the therapist should select a different resource or resource image and determine if it can be successfully installed. The therapist may want to encourage the child to set aside the negative material in an imaginal container before proceeding. In addition, the therapist may choose to use very short sets (three to five saccades) to decrease the possibility of activating negative material.

The therapist should next consider the use of a future template to verify that the resource can indeed assist the child in coping with the initially identified challenging situation.

In future sessions, the therapist should check resources that have been installed as well as the parent's written log for any feedback.

During trauma-focused EMDR desensitization, the therapist may use previously installed resources as interweaves to address blocked responses to treatment. The therapist should be aware that if he or she chooses to use RDI during desensitization, processing of traumatic material has stopped.

Script for Resource Development and Installation for Children

1. Identifying needed resources: *"I want you to think about something that bothers you. It could be something that happened at home or school or with friends. When you think about that thing, how do you want to think or feel about it instead? What would you rather be able to do? What do you think could help you right now to do that? Let's figure out what you might need to be able to feel or act the way you want to."*

2. Resource development: exploring various types of resources (choose one):

    a. Mastery experiences and images: *"Think about a time when you felt _____ [e.g., strong, safe, confident, soothed, able to tolerate your feelings]."* *"Think about a time when you were able to act _____ [e.g., smarter, stronger, calmer, friendlier, etc.]."* *"Tell me about a time when you remember feeling like that or when you acted like that. Can you see yourself tomorrow or next week with that _____ [e.g., stronger feeling, some type of different behavior]."*

    b. Relational resources [models and supportive figures]: *"Think of people or things that would help you feel the way that you want to feel. Can you think of somebody who is like that? These could be real people like your mom or dad, grandparents* [identify significant adults/friends in the child's life] *or these could be people in books or on television that help you feel good. Are there any animals or pets that you think could help you with this?"*

    c. Metaphors and symbolic resources: *"Is there something you can think of that would make you feel _____* [whatever resource it is], *like a magic feather, or sword, magic wand, fairy, or a cool tree house?"* *"Is there anything from your drawings, daydreams, ideas, games you've played, books you like, or movies you've watched?"*

3. Resource development: accessing more information: [Working with one resource image or association at a time]: *"When you think about that _____ [e.g., experience, person, symbol, etc.], what do you see? What do you hear? What do you smell? What do you notice in your body when you think about it?"* Use examples and physical motions to demonstrate for the child. *"What feelings do you notice as you focus on this picture or memory?"* Make verbatim notes of these descriptions to use in the following sections.

4. Checking the resource: *"When you think about that picture _____ [repeat description of image] and the _____ [repeat description of feelings, sensations, smells, sounds, etc.], how does that make you feel?"* Then verify that the selected resource would help the child cope with the challenging situation by asking: *"When you think about _____ [the target situation] how true or helpful does _____ [repeat description of the image and feelings] feel to you now, from 1, not helpful, to 7, completely true or helpful?"* [The therapist uses whatever measurement is most applicable to the individual child and his or her development.]

5. Reflecting the resource: *"Continue to let yourself think about _____ [repeat the description of the picture], and notice the _____."* Repeat descriptions of feelings, sensations, and sounds verbatim and check whether the association is, in fact, positive. Verify whether the child can attend to and tolerate a connection to the resource without negative associations or

affect. Do not continue if the child reports a negative association with this resource, and consider starting over with another resource.

6. Resource installation: *"Now, think about* _____ [repeat the patient's verbatim description of the image and associated emotions and sensations] *and follow my fingers* [or tones, buzzies, lights, taps, etc.]." The therapist then provides several short sets of bilateral stimulation with 4 to 6 complete movements in each set. After each set of bilateral stimulation, the therapist makes a general inquiry. *"What do you get now?"* The bilateral stimulation is not continued if the client reports negative associations or affect. The negative material is either contained imaginally [e.g., in a box, vault, etc.] before proceeding or the process is started over with an alternate resource association.

7. Strengthening the resource: linking with verbal or sensory cues: *"Remember* _____ [mastery resource]. *What can you say about yourself now?" "Imagine that person* [i.e., for relational resources] *standing near you and giving you what you need. Imagine that he or she knows exactly what to say to you. Exactly what you need to hear. Imagine morphing with this person or stepping into his or her body."* Or, *"Imagine holding this*_____ [metaphoric resource] *in your hands. Imagine having this picture or feeling all around you. Take a deep breath and have it all go inside you. Notice where you feel that good feeling in your body. Can you touch it? Can you smell it? Can you taste it?"* Cue the child to access sensory input from all senses. Continue with short sets of BLS as long as processing appears helpful.

8. Cue word or phrase: *"Is there a word or thing to say that we can use for us to remember that thing? What's the best word to help us remember?"* Write the word and check to make sure it fits. *"So if I say* _____ *does it make you think about that thing?"*

    a. Linking cue word or phrase with resource: *"Think about* _____ [repeat the patient's verbatim description of the image and associated emotions and sensations] *and the word* _____ *and follow my fingers* [or tones, buzzies, lights, taps, etc.]." The therapist then provides several short sets of bilateral stimulation with four to six complete movements in each set. After each set of bilateral stimulation, the therapist makes a general inquiry. *"What do you get now?"*

    b. Practicing cue word with disturbance: *"Can you think about something little that happened this last week that bugged you a little bit that you'd like to have that thought or feeling with instead? Let's pretend that you can use that thought or feeling and the word* ____ *to make that little thing stop bugging you now."* The therapist then provides several short sets of bilateral stimulation with four to six complete movements in each set. After each set of bilateral stimulation, the therapist makes a general inquiry. *"What do you get now?"*

9. Establishing a future template: *"If there was something tomorrow, the next day, or next week you'd want to use this thought with, what would it be? Pretend that you're using that thing with all the smells, sounds, and feelings and the word* _____. *Think about that just the way you need to feel it. Now follow my* [fingers, taps, buzzies]." The therapist then provides several short sets of bilateral stimulation with four to six complete movements in each set. After each set of bilateral stimulation, the therapist makes a general inquiry. *"What do you get now?"* Continue with short sets of bilateral stimulation as long as processing improves the resource. This process may be repeated for each of the qualities the patient wants to strengthen. In future sessions,

the therapist should check resources that have been installed as well as the patient's feedback. When the patient is ready for stage two, trauma-focused work, the therapist can begin the session by first bringing in and strengthening (with bilateral stimulation) the resources needed to address the traumatic material. During trauma-focused EMDR reprocessing, the therapist may use previously installed resources as interweaves (Shapiro, 1995, pp. 244–271) to address blocked responses to treatment. However, any use of an interweave is considered only one channel. Processing is not considered complete until the undistorted target is accessed and associated channels are followed to resolution without distortion.

RDI Worksheet—Part 1

Needed resources (qualities, capacities, strengths, needs, feelings, beliefs as identified by client): _____

_____

_____

_____

_____

_____

Resource Development

Mastery experiences and images: _____

_____

_____

_____

_____

_____

Relational resources: _____

_____

_____

_____

_____

_____

Metaphors and symbols: _____

_____

_____

_____

_____

_____

Clinician's Signature:_____Date: _____

After completing this worksheet, the therapist needs to consider the child's needs for further developing the resource. If so, continue with the next section.

RDI Worksheet—Part 2

Needed resource (quality, capacity, strength, need, feeling, belief as identified by client): _____

_____

_____

_____

Resource target selected (e.g., mastery experience or image, supportive person, metaphor, or symbol):

_____

_____

_____

_____

Image: _____

_____

_____

_____

Additional details (sounds, smells, textures, etc.): _____

_____

_____

_____

Positive emotions: _____

_____

_____

_____

Positive physical sensations (location and description): _____

_____

_____

_____

Associated positive cue words: _____

_____

_____

_____

What strengthens the client's connection to the resource (i.e., hearing words of encouragement from a supportive person, holding the resource in their hands, moving closer to the resource)?

_____

_____

_____

Clinician's Signature:_____Date: _____

Abbreviated RDI Protocol

(We included this abbreviated protocol as a checklist to remind the therapist of the steps of RDI.)

Step 1: Identify needed resources (qualities, capacities, strengths, needs, feelings, beliefs as identified by the client).

Step 2: Resource development: exploring various types of resources

Mastery experiences and images

Relational resources

Metaphors and symbols

Step 3: Resource development: accessing more information (working with one resource image at a time)—what do you see, hear, smell, feel (emotions and sensations)?

Step 4: Checking the resource: Check the resource by asking the client to notice how he or she feels when focusing on the resource image. Response must be positive. If not, reevaluate the resource selected.

Step 5: Reflecting the resource.

Step 6: Installing the resource: Install the resource using several short sets of BLS, four to six complete movements in each set. What are you feeling or noticing now?

Step 7: Strengthen the resource by linking with verbal (i.e., positive cue words or words of encouragement from a supportive figure) or sensory cues (i.e., feel the supportive figure's hand on your shoulder, breathe in that energy).

Step 8: Cue word or phrase.

Linking cue word or phrase with resource

Practicing cue word or phrase with disturbance

Step 9: Establish a future template.

Mapping and Graphing for Use in EMDR With Children

This section is included in chapter 5 of the book, *EMDR and the Art of Psychotherapy With Children.* The Mapping and Graphing tools were designed by the authors to help organize the EMDR protocol especially with children and can be integrated into the eight-phase protocol from the beginning with Client History and Treatment Planning.

Introduction to Mapping and Graphing

Mapping and Graphing are tools for organizing targets, resources, and mastery experiences for children. We created these techniques in order to assist clients in their ability to grasp the concepts associated with EMDR through art therapy in a tangible clinical process. Throughout EMDR treatment, Mapping and Graphing are tangible ways to conceptualize the work to be done in treatment and then to reevaluate treatment progress and outcomes. Both techniques teach children to self-assess and enhance their metacognitive skills or their ability to think about their thoughts and feelings while having new tools to explain their experiences. Finally, both Mapping and Graphing can be used as containers where children can have any distressing memories or emotions stick to the paper until the disturbance can be resolved.

Instructions to the Therapist for Mapping

Mapping targets for EMDR is a technique utilized to organize the information collected when preparing for processing a client's issues with EMDR. Initially Mapping was used to organize the child client's trauma history in order to identify targets for EMDR; however, after using the process on a regular basis we found that Mapping targets is an effective tool for utilization when proceeding with the full EMDR protocol for clients of all ages. This protocol is written specifically for children but can also be used very effectively with adults. The therapist can use Mapping for case conceptualization beginning during the Client History and Treatment Planning Phases and continue through the entire eight phases of the EMDR protocol. Mapping integrates with the specific steps of the protocol and helps clients understand the conceptualization that the therapist might consider. Mapping helps to elucidate how EMDR works in a tangible manner for even the youngest clients.

As the therapist begins to explore the parameters of the problem based on parent input and discussion with the child, data regarding the client's trauma history begins to arise and the therapist explains to the client that this is all important information that we need to pay attention to in order to help their brain fix the problem. The therapist can suggest to the child that talking about this information may bother them a little; therefore, with their assistance the therapist would like to create a map where they can put all the important parts about their worries or fears. The therapist can suggest to the child that by putting their worries on the paper, they might not have to worry as much, because the map can be used as a container. The therapist shows the child that they are going to use a piece of paper and pen to begin to make a map of things that bother them and the therapist needs the child's help to get the map correct. The therapist suggests that the child can help with the map or do it entirely by himself or herself.

After completing the map, explain to the child that the map can be changed at any time if something has been forgotten or if something changes. Finally, it is important to encourage the child to take ownership of the map and explain that he or she is in charge of what happens next with the map.

Session Protocol for Mapping

1. The therapist greets the child and parent in the waiting room and escorts them to the therapist's office.

2. The therapist reviews the previous session and answers any questions from the child and parent.

3. The therapist assesses general functioning since the previous session. The therapist reviews the current status of any symptoms identified in the previous session and explores any new symptoms. *"Has anything changed since our last session?"* Ask both the child and the parent. (Refer to the book for detailed instructions.)

4. The therapist reviews any notations from the parent on the Child/Adolescent Symptom Monitoring Form.

5. The therapist reminds the child of the Safe/Calm Place and Stop Signal.

6. Interview the parent about identifying possible targets for EMDR.

7. Interview the child about identifying targets for EMDR and compare with parents' responses.

8. Explain Mapping to the child.

9. Begin drawing the map. Have the child pick single words to put in the figure on the map that will help to identify what worry is in each shape.

10. Review Safe/Calm Place or use Cognitive Interweaves as needed if the child becomes anxious while identifying targets.

11. Teach the child how map figures can also be used as containers where targets stay stuck to the map.

12. Remind the child that the map can be added to or changed at any time.

13. Ask the child to help rank the targets on the map.

14. Do SUD for targets on the map.

15. Review the SUD compared to the ranking.

16. Explain how targets get connected in the brain. Draw lines between targets on the map and show the strength of the connection by the thickness of the line.

17. Ask what is the bad thought for each target.

18. Ask what is the good thought for each target.

19. Assess the VoC for each target.

20. Identify the feeling associated with each target.

21. Identify links between targets/feelings for the child.

22. Assess for feeder memories that are associated with the same feeling.

23. Have the child choose a target to start with and point out associations with other targets including similar feelings and body sensations.

24. Desensitize targets and reevaluate the map.

25. Continue with the next target.

Script for Mapping Targets

Per the protocol and scripts already included in this book, start with Client History and Treatment Planning. Focus on attunement with the child and listening for negative cognitions and possible targets for EMDR processing. It is helpful for the therapist to make notes of the client's negative cognitions and potential targets.

In the Preparation Phase the therapist explains EMDR to parents *and* to children.

Then the therapist assesses the parent's current stability and ability to participate in the EMDR process with the child.

Teach Safe/Calm Place to child. During this process allow the child to experiment with the different types of bilateral stimulation: tapping, drumming, stomping, using the buzzies, and so on.

Teach the Stop Signal.

Interview the parent about identifying possible targets for EMDR.

Interview the child about identifying targets for EMDR and compare with parents' responses.

Explain Mapping to the child. *"I would like you to help me create a map where we put all of your worries, owies, etc. Do you know what a map is?"* If the child knows what a map is, continue with the Mapping process. If not, explain what a map is to the child. *"Today we will start your map that shows where the things that bother you or the worries that you have are, just like in your head* (therapist can point to his or her own head and the child's head). *Today we are starting with the map, but we can change it or add worries to it at anytime. Remember that it is your brain that will fix your worries and that I can teach you a way to help your brain shrink the worries and even make the worries go away."*

With large drawing paper and pen or pencil draw a large odd shape in the middle of the paper and ask the child to identify his or her biggest worry to start the map. *"On this paper, I want us to start drawing your map by picking the biggest worry that you have or the thing that is bothering you the most right now."* Help the child to write his or her biggest concern or symptom in the shape in order to begin the map. Have the child pick single words to put in the figure on the map that will help to identify what worry is in each shape.

"When we make the map you might feel a little bit scared or worried, but remember you're safe here in my office and if you get too scared you can always practice using your safe place like we learned before. Do you remember how to use your safe place to feel better?" If needed, review Safe/Calm Place or continue identifying targets.

In addition to Safe/Calm Place, you can teach the child to use the figures on the map as containers. *"Do you see this big worry here on your map? What do we need to do to keep that worry locked into that shape on the map so it won't bother you?"* Usually children are very creative and come up with many ideas, but you can assist as necessary. You might want to suggest to the child that the shape on the map can have steel walls with lasers to keep anything from escaping the shape. You can also add, *"When we put your worry onto the map, we're sealing it into the shape so it won't come off and bother you. It will stay stuck on the map until we take it off to shrink it. Is that ok with you?"* Continue to collect targets by asking the child to identify more things that bother them, and suggest things that the child's parent may have identified as well. For instance, you may say to Johnny, *"Your mom thinks that you get in trouble a lot in school because you are mad about your daddy leaving. Do you think this is something we should put on your map?"* Continue by asking Johnny if there are things that his mom doesn't understand or know about that should also be on his map. Continue with Mapping all of the child's worries by adding to the drawing. You can add additional pieces of paper as needed to identify all of the child's worries. Sometimes this process proceeds very quickly and you can move to the next phases of the EMDR protocol, while other times this process takes an entire session. If you note that the child is becoming agitated in completing the Mapping, you can offer cognitive interweaves, suggest that the child practice his Safe/Calm Place, or stop and conduct a resource installation in order for the child to cope with Mapping targets. See chapters on cognitive interweaves for children and resource installation for children. Throughout the remainder of this process, try to become attuned with the child and use the child's language regarding how the child labels whatever problems or worries he or she has.

Continue to identify other worries to add to the map. Engage the child in helping you create the map or let the child create the map as appropriate for the child's developmental level and understanding.

Explain to the child that you will also be writing notes, because what she or he says is very important and you want to make sure you remember it correctly. *"I am writing down what you are telling me because it is very important and I'm old and I don't want to forget what you are telling me. Is that ok with you?"*

When the child has identified all the worries that he or she wants to put on the map for the day, remind the child that he or she can add to the map at any time. *"Remember we can change the map at any time if we've forgotten something or something changes."*

Next ask the child to help rank the targets on the map. *"Now I want you to help me know which worry is the biggest or bothers you the most. Would you show me which one is the biggest or worst?"* Proceed with the ranking process from worst or bothers me the most until littlest worry or *"It doesn't bother me hardly at all."*

After completing the ranking process, explain SUD to the child and ask the child to identify a SUD for each target on the map. *"I want us to be able to tell how much something bothers you so when I ask you to tell me how much something bothers you, we can use numbers or you can show me with your hands like this."* The therapist demonstrates SUD based on the distance between the therapist's hands. The therapist then says. *"Is it this big, this big, or this big?"* The therapist can also use other measurements for the SUD. SUD can be bigger than the whole world or universe or deeper than the ocean, or the therapist can ask the child to tell what the biggest thing is that he or she can imagine. After that the therapist asks the child for the smallest thing they can imagine. Then the therapist asks the child to tell how big each worry is for each target on the map and this is noted on the map. *"What's the biggest thing you can think of in the whole world?"* Whatever the child answers, the therapist explains, *"That tells me that your worry would bother you a lot if it's as big as _____ (repeat child's answer)."* The therapist then asks the child, *"What's the smallest thing you could imagine?"* Whatever the child answers, the therapist says *"That tells me that your worry doesn't bother you at all if it's as small as _____ (repeat child's answer). "That's how we will both know how much something bothers you."*

When I do this process, because I'm (R.T.) already working with a map metaphor, sometimes I will ask the child to show me how big the worry is on the map or globe. I will say things like *"Is it as big as Arizona or bigger?"* (We live in Arizona). If it's bigger than Arizona, I say, *"Maybe it's as big as the whole United States or bigger?"* If it's bigger than the whole United States we continue with as big as the whole world, the whole universe, or "infinity and beyond." Be creative and help the child feel validated in how big the worry is for them.

After completing the SUD, review the SUD compared to the ranking. The therapist notes if the SUD and ranking do not match as a way to assure that the child is understanding the concept of assessing how distressful the target is for them.

After completing SUD, the therapist also uses the map as a way to explain how worries or memories get connected in our brains. *"In our brains sometimes memories or worries get connected. Like you told me that when you think about your dad you are sad and when you think about your dog dying you get sad. On your map let's show how strong you think the connection is between the worries."* The therapist demonstrates to the child how to draw lines between the worries and then can make the line very thick or thin depending on how big the child thinks the connection is between the two targets. This serves to help the child understand how his or her brain works and why when feeling sad the child thinks of his or her dad and his or her dog. In addition to being educational for the child, we are also creating links that will ideally assist in linking the two memories when we proceed with desensitization.

After the SUD, ask the child to help the therapist understand what the bad thought is that goes with the memory. *"When you think about that worry, what's the bad thought that goes with that worry?"* If necessary offer suggestions or use the "Kids' List of Cognitions." Then ask the child what they would like to think instead or *"What's the good thought?"*

After identifying NC and PC, assess for a VoC. The therapist can use the example of the VoC Bridge by saying, *"If we put your bad thought here* (put bad thought on the left side of the paper) *and your good thought here* (write the good thought on the right side of the paper) *and we make a bridge with seven steps from your bad thought to your good thought* (therapist draws seven steps on an imaginary bridge between the bad thought and the good thought), *where do you think you are right now?"*

After the VoC, ask the child to tell the therapist what the feeling is that goes with the target. Sometimes the therapist may need to offer words for feelings to assist the child. *"When you think of that thing that bothers you and the bad thought, what feelings do you have about that?"*

Once we've identified feelings for the particular memory, look for links between targets for the child. Explain to the child that sometimes things bother us more than we expect because the feeling is connected to something else that bothered us before. For example, if Johnny has identified anger as a feeling associated with one of his targets, ask Johnny to identify other targets where he also might have felt angry and ask if he thinks those are connected to each other. Finally, this may also assist in identifying other feeder memories that are associated with feeling sad, mad, or other feelings.

After identifying the feeling, ask the child where they feel that feeling in their body. Sometimes the child can point and tell you where they feel the worry, while other times we need to take a break and teach mindfulness. *"When you think about that thing that bothers you and the _____ feeling, where do you feel that in your body? Some people feel it in their heads, some people feel it in their hearts, some people feel it in their tummies, and some people feel it in their legs and feet."* The therapist can point to different parts of their body to demonstrate where the child might feel the disturbance.

Once the child has identified the body sensation, the therapist can then explain, *"This map helps to tell us what we need to work on to help you with _____* (repeat child's concerns, symptoms, or behavioral problems). *Each time we work together we will chose something on your map to work on until we can cross all of these off of your map. Do you have any questions?"* Wait for response. *"Let's pick the first thing we want to work on today or next week"* (depending on the amount of time remaining in the session).

Each session the therapist can check in with the child to ask if any changes have occurred that would suggest something or should be added or removed from the map.

Instructions to the Therapist for Graphing

Graphing is a multifaceted technique for elucidating various steps in the EMDR protocol. Graphing involves the therapist teaching the child to use a simple bar graph for identifying and assessing mastery experiences, targets, or symptoms; or evaluating progress in treatment; and/or as a container. The purpose for Graphing is to help the child develop the observer self and to have a concrete technique for understanding and documenting the pieces of the EMDR treatment protocol.

Graphing for mastery experiences is used for the purpose of identifying resources, activities, abilities, and experiences that have created a positive experience for the child. For example, Riley feels good about how far he hit the ball in his baseball game. Riley would then note hitting the baseball as a mastery experience on his graph. The use of identifying and Graphing mastery experiences provides the child with positive associations to the EMDR process, as well as developing a positive internal scaffolding in preparation for the desensitization phase.

For target and symptom identification, Graphing helps the child create a list of his problems, worries, or "bothers" through drawing them in a concrete, visual manner. The purpose of Graphing targets assists both the therapist and the child in selecting which targets should be reprocessed first.

As an evaluation tool, Graphing can be used at the end of the session or for reevaluation in the following session. After the child has identified either resources or targets, the child and therapist can measure the strength of the resource or the level of competency over the target and then reevaluate progress. Graphing is not used as a SUD scale.

Graphing can also be used as a container during or at the end of the session if the child is flooded by disturbing emotions. The therapist can instruct the child to have worries or bothers stay on the paper like a container.

The therapist can have the child make different graphs for each type of Graphing technique, or some of the graphs can be combined. Graphing is a fluid and ongoing part of the treatment protocol in EMDR.

Session Protocol for Graphing

1. The therapist greets the child and parent in the waiting room and escorts them to the therapist's office.

2. The therapist reviews the previous session and answers any questions from the child and parent.

3. The therapist assesses general functioning since the previous session. The therapist reviews the current status of any symptoms identified in the previous session and explores any new symptoms. *"Has anything changed since our last session?"* Ask both the child and the parent. (Refer to the book for detailed instructions.)

4. The therapist reviews any notations from the parent on the Child/Adolescent Symptom Monitoring Form.

5. The therapist reminds the child of the Safe/Calm Place and Stop Signal.

6. Interview the parent about identifying possible targets for EMDR.

7. Interview the child about identifying targets for EMDR and compare with the parent's responses.

8. Explain Graphing to the child using the following script to identify first resources and mastery experiences.

9. Use Graphing to identify targets using the script. If necessary, remind the child of Safe/Calm Place if the child becomes anxious while identifying targets.

10. Pick one target to continue with the Assessment Phase of EMDR (see section 3 of this book) using the pieces of the protocol.

11. At the end of the session use Graphing for assessing progress in treatment and remind the child that the graph can also serve as a container.

12. Review the mastery graph as a resource for the child to use between sessions as needed.

13. At the next session, review the mastery graph before moving to the target graph to continue with the EMDR protocol.

Script for Graphing

First the therapist explores whether the child understands the concept of a graph. Often children as young as 6-years-old have already learned about simple bar graphs in school. Many times, even a 4-year-old can draw a rudimentary graph with a therapist's help. If the child has not heard of a graph, educate him or her to the idea by saying something like, *"I'm going to show you how to draw a graph. A graph is a way to measure things. Today we are going to measure things that you feel good about and things that you think are problems or worries or bothers."*

The therapist demonstrates what a graph is by drawing a large *L* with a crayon on a piece of drawing paper. The therapist divides the vertical line with 10 small, evenly spaced lines to indicate percentages. At the bottom of the vertical line the therapist puts a 0 and in increments of 10, at each line, writes 10%, 20%, and so on, with the top of the line showing 100%. *"This line is how we can measure things with numbers where 0 is we don't feel good about them at all and 100 is where we feel really good about something."*

On the bottom horizontal line the therapist can write or draw examples of either mastery experiences/activities or problems and worries that a child might identify for the graph.

For mastery the therapist says, *"We are going to make a list of the things that you feel good about on the bottom so we can measure them. Can you tell me something you feel really good about?"* The Mastery (or Good Things) Graph can be used in every session. To make a Mastery Graph you ask the child to tell you something that they feel like they do well, or something that makes them feel good about themselves, and list those items at the bottom of the horizontal line in one- or two-word descriptions. *"Can you tell me something else that makes you feel good?"* After collecting mastery experiences, the therapist then asks the child to draw and color in a line vertically that goes up to or as close to 100% as possible. *"Can you draw a line that shows how good you feel about that thing? Ten percent is you feel a little bit good and 50% is you feel pretty good, and 100% is you feel the best about that thing."* The 100% represents how good they feel about the experience or activity. For instance, if Phoebe feels good about her drawing and art, we draw a line from the bottom of the horizontal line all the way up to 100%, meaning she feels as good as she can about her drawing. Then we identify several other activities that she feels positive about and she draws the line somewhere from 0 to 100%, demonstrating how good Phoebe feels about those positive experiences.

Then we install the mastery experience by having the child choose one of these positive experiences and enhance the good feelings in his or her body with bilateral stimulation, similar to the abbreviated RDI protocol. The therapist says to the child, *"So I want you to think about how good that* (mastery experience) *feels in your body and hold on to the buzzies for a second."* The therapist can use whatever type of BLS the child had chosen to install the mastery experience.

When completing a Targeting (or Worries and Problems) Graph, use a separate piece of paper and again have them make an L-shaped graph with percentages on the vertical axis, and list on the bottom the child's reported problems, worries, or bothers. The child then draws a bar or line that represents how much better or more competent the child feels regarding that target, with 100% demonstrating that the problem is resolved and/or the child feels competent to handle the problem or issue. Zero means that the child feels unable to handle the problem at all. *"Now we're going to make a worries or problems graph and we're gonna put all your worries or things that bother you on the bottom and this is how we're going to measure how good you feel about that problem. When it gets to the top or 100% you know you can handle the problem. It's kind of like a report card where we know you can handle that thing and it doesn't bother you or worry you anymore."*

The therapist can then refer back to targets on the graph at the end of a session, to assess the target. *"Ok, so we've worked on this problem, and where do you feel you are with handling that problem now?"* The child can draw the bar upward toward 100%, showing how much better he or she feels regarding the target. Often when one target is resolved, the child will spontaneously report that other targets are resolved. The child can then draw lines on the graph representing how much better they feel about each target.

The graph is also very useful to use in the next session to reevaluate the targets. The therapist says, *"Well, do you remember what we worked on last time? Let's take out our graph and look at it now. So with that problem we worked on, where are you now?"* The child may have increased feelings of competency with handling the problem and the percentage goes up, or occasionally the child is more worried about the problem, so the therapist can give the child a black crayon or marker to show that his or her feelings of competency over the problem actually went down. Children often feel empowered by the process of Graphing because they can see their progress.

The Targeting Graph can also be used as a container at the end of sessions to assist the child in not having strong emotions or acting out behaviors between sessions. The therapist can simply say, *"This is your worry or bother graph and we're leaving them here on this paper in my office today. If for any reason these problems bother you when you go home, then you can imagine putting them back on the graph in my office and leaving them here."*

There are variations on Graphing and we encourage you to use your own ideas to adapt the graph to your own client's needs after you have practiced the basic concept.

Section 12

Future Template for Use in EMDR With Children

This section relates to chapter 7 of the book, *EMDR and the Art of Psychotherapy With Children.*

Instructions to the Therapist for Future Template

This is different than Future Template for adults, in that children need immediate and current positive behavioral actions to take, because it is empowering to them. Therefore, once earlier memories and present triggers and symptoms are adequately resolved regarding the specific target, the therapist explores how the child would rather feel and act in the future. The therapist may have to teach the skills to the child (e.g., social skills, assertiveness, anger management).

Sometimes a therapist will not have enough time to complete this Future Template process all in one session. If time is limited, the therapist should omit Future Template at this point and proceed with Closure in order to complete the session. If Future Template is omitted, the therapist should return to the Future Template process in the next session immediately after completing Reevaluation.

Sometimes when reprocessing a target, the progression of the session will move logically from the initial target to the future and the therapist can have the child imagine successfully implementing the future desired behavior related to the target. For example, if the child presented for therapy with a symptom of not being able to sleep in his or her own bed, the therapist would identify past experiences and events impacting this issue and then resolve current issues before moving to the future in which the child imagines successfully sleeping in his or her own bed. The child's future success and mastery of this issue is installed with BLS; however, some children will experience anticipatory anxiety about the future desired behavior and then the therapist will need to complete the entire Assessment Protocol to target that future event. The ultimate goal of the Future Template is for the child to have a positive template for the future and to leave the therapy session feeling competent to handle the specific issue.

Session Protocol for Future Template

1. The therapist greets the child and parent in the waiting room and escorts them to the therapist's office.

2. The therapist reviews the previous session and answers any questions from the child and parent.

3. The therapist assesses general functioning since the previous session. The therapist reviews the current status of any symptoms identified in the previous session and explores any new symptoms. *"Has anything changed since our last session?"* Ask both the child and the parent. (Refer to the book for detailed instructions.)

4. The therapist reviews any notations from the parent on the Child/Adolescent Symptom Monitoring Form.

5. The therapist explains Future Template using the following script, completing as much of the process as possible given the time available in the session.

6. The therapist follows the protocol for closing the session, explains the Child/Adolescent Symptom Monitoring Form for use between sessions, and gives the parent a copy of the Child/Adolescent Symptom Monitoring Form for parent use.

7. The therapist reviews treatment goals with the child and parent, answers any questions, and reminds the child and parent of resources for use between sessions.

8. The therapist schedules the next appointment.

9. The therapist escorts the child and parent to the waiting room/exit.

Future Template Script

Target: *"What would you like to be able to do?"* The response should be a positive behavior like "Sleep in my own bed."

NC/PC/VoC: *"When you think about that thing you'd like to be able to do, what's the bad thought?"* The therapist identifies a new NC for future action. The therapist then asks the child, *"What would you rather tell yourself instead,"* or the therapist explains, *"What's the good thought?"* Then the therapist elicits the VoC for the new PC by asking, *"When you think about that thing you want to be able to do and those words* [therapist repeats PC] *how true does that seem to you right now, from 1, completely false or not true, to 7, completely true?"*

Emotion: The therapist continues by identifying the emotion, saying to the child, *"When you think about that thing you wanna be able to do, what's the feeling that goes with that?"*

SUD: The therapist continues by identifying the SUD, by saying to the child, *"How disturbing does that feel?"*

Body Sensation: The therapist then identifies body sensation by asking, *"Where do you feel that in your body?"* [The therapist can use examples of body sensations as discussed previously.]

Once the therapist has elicited the future target, NC/PC, VoC, emotion, SUD, and body sensation for future desired behaviors/actions/feelings, the therapist continues by saying *"Sometime in the next day or so, I want you to think about* _____ [the desired positive behavior, e.g., sleeping in my own bed alone, handling anger in an appropriate way] *with those words* _____ [say the new positive cognition] *with all the* _____ [elicit positive visual cues], _____ [positive sounds], _____ [and positive kinesthetic sensations]." The therapist processes Future Template with BLS—24 saccades. If something negative comes up then process the negative through with whatever comes up as the target. If the adaptive resolution continues in a positive direction, continue as follows.

> *"Now, I want you to imagine* [or pretend] *three nights from now with the same* _____ [desired positive behavior]." Do BLS.

> *"Now in 1 week, . . .* [same words and scenario]." Do BLS.

> *"Now in 1 month, . . .* [same words and scenario]." Do BLS.

> *"Now let's pretend we are seeing yourself when you're bigger and one time when you would need* _____ [desired behavior]. *Imagine the* _____ [positive behavior] *and* [positive words] _____ [PC]." Do BLS.

You can have the child draw a picture, use the sand tray, or make a clay sculpture at any point. Stay attuned to evaluate any negative associations or distortions that may emerge. The child should feel emotionally, physically, and cognitively comfortable with the anticipated event.

Section 13

Assessing Fidelity or Adherence to the EMDR Protocol With Child Clients

This section relates to chapter 1 of the book, *EMDR and the Art of Psychotherapy With Children.*

Instructions to the Therapist for Assessing Fidelity or Adherence to the EMDR Protocol With Child Clients

Assessing fidelity or adherence to the EMDR protocol is important for a variety of reasons, both for clinical purposes and for research purposes. It is important for a treating therapist to assess fidelity in clinical practice in order to ensure that the therapist is using the complete EMDR protocol without omitting important words, procedural steps, or phases of the protocol. By using a Fidelity Questionnaire, the therapist can monitor his or her own adherence to the protocol in order to improve practice and prevent therapist drift.

For research purposes, adherence to the protocol is important in order that researchers reporting on the efficacy of EMDR can explain exactly what therapists did in order to call the treatment EMDR. The goal of the fidelity study is to create greater understanding of behavioral change as well as to develop interventions to promote change (Rounsville, Carroll, and Onken, 2001). In spite of the positive treatment outcomes reported in the studies of EMDR with adult clients, methodological concerns have contributed to a mixed response to the assessment of the efficacy of EMDR. Maxfield and Hyer (2002) concluded that research on EMDR treatment outcomes is affected by the methodological structures of the individual study. At the root of variable outcomes in studies of EMDR are differences in number of subjects, treatment fidelity, and number of treatment sessions, with few studies mentioning fidelity to the EMDR protocol. By documenting precision in the treatment protocol, researchers can support the efficacy of the treatment protocol rather than contributing treatment outcome to extraneous variables. In addition, fidelity is also imperative to research in order that the research study can be replicated.

We recommend that therapists continue to conduct self-assessment of treatment fidelity in order to demonstrate adherence to the EMDR protocol and improve clinical skills. Therapists who make any changes to the protocol or omit any pieces of the protocol should document their clinical decision making for the modification

99

or deletions. We have included a progress note for therapists to note clinical decision making during EMDR. The forms were included to teach therapists to monitor fidelity to EMDR protocol while also noting clinical decisions if deviations from the protocol were necessary. The Fidelity Questionnaire can be used for self review or in consultation.

Furthermore, in order to encourage therapists to conduct regular self-assessment we have included a Fidelity Questionnaire. This questionnaire is used to determine whether the therapist completed all the phases of the protocol and procedural steps.

Finally, the progress note and Fidelity Questionnaire can be used for peer consultation or for consultation for certification.

Following the Fidelity Questionnaire, we have included references for pre- and post-treatment assessment tools. We encourage therapists to use standardized assessment forms to measure symptom presentation at the onset of therapy and treatment outcome throughout and at the conclusion of the treatment regime.

EMDR Therapist Assessment of Fidelity to Treatment Model Form

Client name: _____ Therapist: _____

Session date: _____ Session #: _____ Client ID: _____

To be completed by the therapist after every therapy session.

1) Did you run into any challenges implementing the treatment method?

___Yes ___ No   If yes, please describe the nature of the difficulties.

_____

_____

_____

_____

_____

_____

_____

_____

_____

_____

_____

_____

_____

_____

2) Did you have to make any adaptations to the protocol? ___ Yes ___ No
If yes, please document the adaptations and why they were necessary (if reason for adaptation was noted in #1, just state "see #1").

_____

_____

_____

_____

_____

_____

_____

_____

_____

_____

_____

_____

_____

_____

_____

_____

Therapist signature: _____ Date: _____

EMDR Fidelity Questionnaire

Phase 1: Client History and Treatment Planning

Did you identify a client history and treatment planning process?   ❑ YES   ❑ NO

Phase 2: Preparation

Did you identify aspects of the therapist preparing the client for additional phases of the EMDR protocol?   ❑ YES   ❑ NO

Phase 3: Assessment

Did you identify aspects of the therapist conducting assessment of the client in anticipation of proceeding with Phase 4 Desensitization?   ❑ YES   ❑ NO

Did the therapist identify a specific memory or picture and then identify the worst part?   ❑ YES   ❑ NO

If yes, please describe the target._____

Did you identify a NC?   ❑ YES   ❑ NO

If yes, please describe the NC. _____

Did you identify a PC?   ❑ YES   ❑ NO

If yes, please describe the PC. _____

Did you identify a VoC?   ❑ YES   ❑ NO

If yes, what was the initial VoC?_____

Did you identify an emotion?   ❑ YES   ❑ NO

If yes, what was the emotion identified?_____

Did the therapist get a SUD?_____   ❑ YES   ❑ NO

Did you identify a body sensation?   ❑ YES   ❑ NO

If yes, what body sensation was identified?_____

Phase 4: Desensitization

Did the therapist desensitize the target to SUD of 0 and VoC of 7?   ❑ YES   ❑ NO

If no, did the therapist proceed with desensitization and process an incomplete session?   ❑ YES   ❑ NO   ❑ NA

Phase 5: Installation

Did you identify the therapist utilizing an installation process?
❑ YES   ❑ NO

Phase 6: Body Scan

Did you identify the therapist proceeding with the body scan process?
❑ YES   ❑ NO

Phase 7: Closure

Did you identify the therapist implementing a closure process?
❑ YES   ❑ NO

Phase 8: Reevaluation

At some point in the client's treatment, did you identify a revaluation process utilized with the client?   ❑ YES   ❑ NO

Three-pronged protocol:

1. Was there evidence that the therapist assessed processing in the present?
    ❑ YES   ❑ NO

2. Was there evidence that the therapist assessed processing in the present?
    ❑ YES   ❑ NO

3. Was there evidence of the therapist's application of Future Template by guiding the client through application of new skills to a future event?   ❑ YES   ❑ NO

Conclusions

For many years, therapists have discussed the challenges of treating young children with the full EMDR protocol. Because EMDR is based on the ability to abstract, which theoretically does not develop until late childhood and early adolescence, the EMDR protocol needed to be translated into developmentally appropriate language for young children. Our research study (in our book, *EMDR and The Art of Psychotherapy With Children*) indicated that the child's lack of ability to abstract does not have to interfere with the therapist's ability to use the full EMDR protocol. The therapist needs to offer bridges and translations for the child to understand the abstract concepts of EMDR. Since some procedural steps of the EMDR protocol are more difficult to elicit with children, we decided to write a treatment manual to translate the procedural steps into specific techniques for processing with children without omitting any pieces of the protocol. Eliciting the eight phases of the EMDR protocol is anything but a linear process with children; however, the challenges of using the protocol with children do not mean that the protocol cannot be used. For example, children clearly needed different resources than adolescents and adults to communicate the pieces of the EMDR protocol. Children were much less likely to produce all the phases of the protocol verbally but instead were successful with expressive techniques, including play therapy and art therapy. Offering alternative methods for expression did not preclude the therapist from demonstration of fidelity to the eight phases.

Therapists may benefit from specialty training and tools to demonstrate fidelity to the EMDR protocol with young children. Through the use of a written treatment manual to guide adherence to the EMDR protocol with children, along with consultation and support, therapists are given creative tools for adhering to the EMDR protocol with young children. Preliminary findings from research being conducted by the authors document that the full protocol can be used with even young children.

By studying the book, *EMDR and the Art of Psychotherapy With Children*, and using the protocols and scripts included in this treatment manual, therapists can improve their practice in treating even the youngest of clients with EMDR. The ultimate goal is to document that EMDR is an efficacious and evidence-based practice for the treatment of children when therapists can learn to use the protocol in developmentally adjusted practice.

References

Adler-Tapia, R. L. (2000). *Traumatic stress symptom checklist for infants, toddlers, and preschoolers.* Unpublished, available from the author.

Adler-Tapia, R. L., & Settle, C. S. (2008). *EMDR and the art of psychotherapy with children.* New York: Springer Publishing.

Armstrong, J. G., Putnam, F. W., Carlson, E. B., Libero, D. Z., & Smith, S. R. (1997). Development and validation of a measure of adolescent dissociation: The Adolescent Dissociative Experiences Scale. *Journal of Nervous and Mental Disorders, 185*(8), 491–497.

Briere, J. (1996). *Trauma Symptom Checklist for Children (TSCC) professional manual.* Odessa, FL: Psychological Assessment Resources.

Korn, D. L., & Leeds, A.M. (2002). Preliminary evidence of efficacy for EMDR resource development and installation in the stabilization phase of treatment of complex posttraumatic stress disorder. *Journal of Clinical Psychology, 58*(12), 1465–1487.

Maxfield, L., & Hyer, L. (2002). The relationship between efficacy and methodology studies investigating EMDR treatment of PTSD. *Journal of Clinical Psychology, 58*(1), 23–41.

Putnam, F. W. (1997). *Dissociation in children and adolescents: A developmental perspective.* New York: Guilford.

Reynolds, C. R., & Kamphaus, R. W. (2004). *Behavioral assessment system for children* (2nd ed.). Bloomington, MN: Pearson Education, Inc.

Rounsaville, B. J., Carroll, K. M., & Onken, L. S. (2001, Summer). A stage model of behavioral therapies research: Getting started and moving on from stage 1. *Clinical Psychology: Science and Practice, 8*(2), 133–142.

Shapiro, F. (1995). *Eye movement desensitization and reprocessing: Basic principles, protocols, and procedures.* New York: Guilford Press.

Shapiro, F. (2001). *Eye movement desensitization and reprocessing: Basic principles, protocols, and procedures* (2nd ed.). New York: Guilford Press.

Wolfe, V. V., Gentile, C., Michienzi, T., Sas, L., & Wolfe, D. A. (1991). The Children's Impact of Traumatic Events Scale: A measure of post-sexual abuse PTSD symptoms. *Behavioral Assessment, 13,* 359–383.

Internet Resources

Adler-Tapia, R., & Settle, C. (Author's Web site.) www.emdrkids.com

American Academy of Child and Adolescent Psychiatry. (1998). *Practice parameters for the assessment and treatment of children and adolescents with posttraumatic stress disorder.* Retrieved February 8, 2008, from http://www.aacap.org/galleries/PracticeParameters/PTSDT.pdf

Association for the Study and Development of Community. *Measures of child social–emotional, behavioral, and developmental well-being, exposure to violence, and environment.* Retrieved September 26, 2007, from http://www.capacitybuilding.net/Measures%20of%20CEV%20and%20outcomes.pdf

Child and adolescent trauma measures. (2007). Retrieved February 8, 2008, from http://origin.web.fordham.edu/images/academics/graduate_schools/gsss/catm%20-%20introduction.pdf

Dr. Bruce Perry's Web site (Child Trauma Web site.): www: childtrauma.org

Emotional Literacy workbooks for kids with free downloads. http://www.kidseq.com/activity.php

International Society for the Study of Dissociation. (2004). Guidelines for the evaluation and treatment of dissociative symptoms in children and adolescents. *Journal of Trauma & Dissociation, 5*(3), Article 10.1300/J229v05n03_09. Retrieved February 8, 2008, from http://www.isst-d.org/education/ChildGuidelines-ISSTD-2003.pdf

National Alliance on Mental Illness. www.nami.org

National Center for PTSD. www.ncptsd.va.gov/ncmain/information/

http://www.nami.org/Content/Microsites191/NAMI_Oklahoma/Home178/Veterans3/Veterans_
Articles/9childrenofveteransandadultswithPTSD.pdf (This is a hand-out on children of veterans and adults with PTSD.)

PTSD and Dissociative Measures for Children. (This site includes all the measures to assess trauma and dissociation for children with free, downloadable copies of the forms.) http://www.podcastforteachers.org/childrenfirstwebsite/cfresources/ptsd_dissociative_measures_201.pdf

Steiner, C. (2002). *Emotional literacy: Intelligence with a heart.* Retrieved February 8, 2008, from http://www.claudesteiner.com/

Training for emotional literacy. http://www.claudesteiner.com/2000_i.htm; Follow links to Steiner's book, *A Warm Fuzzy Tale.*

World Federation for Mental Health. N.I.C.E. Guidelines for treating PTSD. http://www.nice.org.uk/nicemedia/pdf/CG026fullguideline.pdf

Zero to Three Website www.zerotothree.org Website for information on infant toddler development with handouts for parents.

Assessment Tools for Evaluating Children

Researchers will need to determine which assessments tools to use in the study; however, we suggest the CPSS and CRTES be used at minimum for pre/post measures of outcome from the group protocol.

A-DES: Adolescent–Dissociative Experiences Scale (Armstrong, Carlsen, & Putnam, 1997). Retrieved from http://www.energyhealing.net/pdf_files/a-des.pdf

BASC-2: (Behavioral Assessment Scale for Children (2nd ed.). (Reynolds & Kamphaus, 2002.) This form must be purchased.

CDC: Child Dissociative Checklist (CDC), Version 3 (Putnam). Retrieved from http://www.energyhealing.net/pdf_files/cdc.pdf

Child/Adolescent Behavioral Monitoring Form (Adler-Tapia & Settle, 2008).

CITES: Children's Impact of Traumatic Events Scale (Wolfe & Gentile). Retrieved from http://www.swin.edu.au/victims/resources/assessment/ptsd/cites-r.pdf

CPSS: Child PTSD Symptom Scale (Foa, Cashman, Jaycox, & Perry, 1997). Requests for use of this measure must be made to Dr. Edna Foa.

CRTES: *The Child's Reaction to Traumatic Events Scale-Revised* (CRTES-Revised) (Jones, Fletcher, & Ribbe, 2002).

TSCC: Trauma Symptom Checklist for Children (Briere, 1997).

TSSC: Traumatic Stress Symptom Checklist for Infants, Toddlers, and & Preschoolers (Adler-Tapia, 2001). Retrieved from www.emdrkids.com